CONSTITUTIONAL MEDICINE

CONSTITUTIONAL MEDICINE

with especial reference to

THE THREE CONSTITUTIONS
OF
DR VON GRAUVOGL

By

JOHN H. CLARKE, M.D.

GYAN

Published by

GYAN

Gyan Publishing House
5, Ansari Road
Daryaganj, New Delhi-110002
Phone: 011-47034999, 9811692060
E-mail: books@gyanbooks.com

Distribution Network
gyanbooks.com
India, USA, Canada, UK, Australia, France

ISBN : 978-81-212-6693-2 (PB)
First Published, 1930

2nd Impression 2022

Printed at: Gyan Press, Delhi.

CONSTITUTIONAL MEDICINE
Author: JOHN H. CLARKE

CONSTITUTIONAL MEDICINE

with especial reference to

THE THREE CONSTITUTIONS

OF

DR. VON GRAUVOGL

BY

JOHN H. CLARKE, M.D.

"No knowledge is perfect unless it includes an understanding of the origin—that is, the beginning; and as all man's diseases originate in his constitution, it is necessary that his constitution should be known if we wish to know his diseases."—*Paracelsus.*

PREFACE.

Having projected the compilation of a "Repertory of Generalities" it became apparent to me that the work of Dr. von Grauvogl would have to be taken into account, and especially his famous "Constitutions." A reference to such works as I possess, including his *Text-book of Homœopathy* in the American translation by Dr. George W. Shipman, published in 1870, showed me that no process of repertorial condensation could do justice to the subject, and that a complete setting out of it was necessary. As I know of no work of the kind in the English language, and as the subject is of most vital importance not only to Homœopathy but to medicine in general, I have thought well to put it together as best I may, leaving to others to complete what may be lacking in my account of it.

Grauvogl was certainly one of the most remarkable men who were drawn into the Homœopathic fold in the period of its adolescence. For clarity of vision, philosophical and logical mentality, he has no superior. At the same time he was quite in the first rank as a practical physician. He has left on record a series of observations, the parallel of which I have never met. Every one of the cases recorded is a little drama complete in itself, a spring as full of medical wisdom from which every practitioner may draw aceording to his eapacity as it is of human interest. These will all be found in my pages, and to them I have added the eases, no less dramatie and no less vital, of Grauvogl's friend and diseiple, Dr. Bojanus, of Moseow, the ablest of Russian Homœopaths.

Apart from the reeord of clinieal observations whieh it contains, the *Text-book* is not easy reading for moderns. It is in two parts, eaeh part eontaining some 400 pages, and is divided up into numbered paragraphs something after the manner of the *Organon*. This is exeeedingly useful for referenee, but it does not make for eontinuity of thought and reading. Also mueh of the work is neeessarily oecupied with the eurrent medieal doetrines of his day, and these Grauvogl deals with in a spirit of absolute fairness.

The great medieal Panjandrum of Grauvogl's day was Virchow with his " Cellular Pathology " and " Leukæmia," and his dicta had to be taken count of. Grauvogl eorrectly deseribed Virchow as a " politieian and phrase-maker," for Virehow was a leader of Liberals as well as of Medieals. In Grauvogl's view it was not the cell but the moleeule which was the unit of living processes, and on this pereeption his division of the basic eonstitutions of man into three is founded.

Of the human body three-fourths are made up of water—that is of Oxygen and Hydrogen. Carbon and Nitrogen account for most of the remainder. On the eonstant and regular inter-ehange between the tissues and the gases effected by the blood the health of the body depends. On any constant *plus* or *minus* of any of these elements in the blood and tissues depend the basic differences in the constitutions of the individuals so affected. And in these differences —revealed in their symptoms—are found indications for remedies which over-ride indications which might be drawn from the separate symptoms taken independently.

Granvogl's mind was the reverse of everything that savoured of fanaticism or bigotry. His vision was of the *whole*; he did not regard the human organism as made up of independent parts. A born physician, with the genius of cure driving him on, he was compelled to seek and find in Homœopathy the guidance he needed in his search for remedies. But that did not make him abjure all that he had been able to do under the teaching of the physiological or Allopathic school. A man who cannot cure some proportion of his cases with Allopathy is not likely to be very successful in Homœopathy. The physician must be born before he can be made.

In Homœopathy Grauvogl found this supreme merit—it provided a counterfoil or counterpart for comparison with disease-pathology in a drug-pathology which it created. Health, he said, is an abstract idea, disease is something concrete added. Physiological medicine depends on chance experience in isolated cases and experiments on the sick for its progress. As Dr. Dudgeon put it, physiological medicine claims to be orthodox, but it has no "doxy"; it claims to be regular, but it possesses no "rule."

Now that Professor August Bier, of Berlin, has opened the way for a saner attitude towards Homœopathy on the part of the Academies, the work of von Grauvogl should find a welcome in all the Schools. There is no real ground of conflict between the two branches of medicine. It is not a matter of *belief*, it is one of *knowledge*. Either a man knows a certain fact or series of facts, or a certain law and how to use it, or he does not know, and there's an end. It makes no difference to the fact whether it is believed in or not, and disputes about a belief are idle when by taking trouble it is possible to know.

Grauvogl's great achievement consists in his having shown that in prescribing for a patient his constitution often counts for more than the particular complaint in which it manifests itself. He also showed how these different constitutions could be recognised and remedied. Once the constitution is known and cured, all the rest of the symptoms clear up.

This is done in a minor degree by most homœopathic practitioners who have learned from Hahnemann the importance of observing the Conditions under which a symptom occurs or is worse or better; also the Times of recurrence and disappearance, and the Concomitant Symptoms with which it is associated. These particulars, which in general arise from the constitution of the patient and not from the disease from which he is suffering, are often of greater importance than the actual symptoms which they characterise; and it was through patient observance of these that Grauvogl was led to discover the threads running through them.

That the last word has been spoken on this subject by Grauvogl it would be absurd to contend. The modern use of Nosodes by Homœopaths, and of Vaccines and Serums by Allopaths, are instances in which Grauvogl's principles are being carried out in other directions. But nothing new that can be discovered can in any way affect the solid work which Grauvogl has achieved and I feel it a great privilege to be able to set it forth for all to comprehend and use, as I trust it will be found that I have done, in the following pages.

JOHN H. CLARKE.

CONTENTS.

SIGNS USED.

"<" means "worse" or "aggravated by."

">" means "better" or "ameliorated by."

Chapter I

INTRODUCTORY

The following extracts from von Grauvogl's Preface to his *Text-book*, dated "Nuremberg, 1865," will give a clear idea of his aim and object in making that compilation :

Since Homœopathy is nothing but a system of Therapeutics resting on the foundations of all the natural sciences—Chemistry, Physics, Physiology, etc.—a confirmation of the *Organon* and the proof of its conformity with natural science may be required often and at various times. And if the practice of life has a word to say, then it is the duty of every practical physician to make public the knowledge and experience which he has acquired, no matter whether at the present moment these should be regarded favourably or unfavourably; for frequently their real value is finally settled by the future only.

A text-book, however, must present examples ; its principles must be demonstrated and set forth by cases and comparisons taken from life. Then everyone can accurately apply what he has learned to his patient and at the same time confirm it by the test of success. . . .

I resign all pretence to any party stand-point, since there should be no party in science, consequently none in therapeutics. . . .

Aside from its contents as indicated by its title, this work has also the intention to respond to the necessary though not easy demands of a medical logic elucidated by practical examples; for "opinions"—and these, unfortunately, mean nothing but faith in "authorities"— separate physicians into hostile camps and paralyse medical activity which, were it united, would always be attended by the happiest results; these, however, are not attainable under present lamentable circumstances.

The cause of this state of things clearly cannot be in the subjects themselves about which medical factions contend, since these subjects stand to each other in the natural relation of cause and effect, but is brought about by arbitrary "conceptions" thereof. Hence the necessity is abundantly apparent of intertwining the instruments of logic with the contents of a therapeutic text-book.

Those who wish to follow the brilliant logic of Grauvogl's treatise must be referred to the *Text-book* itself. One of my aims will be to "*dis*-intertwine" the practical conclusions from the "intruments of logic" and let the facts speak for themselves. All I will say here is that readers can trust implicitly to Grauvogl's honesty as well as his logic. I will only add this pregnant passage from Part II, page 104 of the *Text-book.* Grauvogl had been citing instances where the teachings of the "physiological school, commonly called Allopathy," were both useful and necessary:

Thus then we must sometimes offer the diseased human organism palliative aid according to the causal law, but as a rule, of course, medical help according to the law of reciprocal action [Homœopathy]. If Homœopathy should seek to treat all cases and every case simply and solely according to the law of similarity, it would fall into the same error as Allopathy. Hence *these sciences are no contrasts in the sense of opposition but rather complements of each other.*

This is an extremely important observation and it is purely from the want of the recognition of this truth that there was ever any opposition to Hahnemann and his teaching. Homœopathy was simply an addition to the knowledge of medical truth and should have been accepted at that. If it was incidentally the means of exploding many cherished medical "opinions" not founded on facts, then the "opinions" ought to have been allowed to pass into the limbo into which all such will eventually have to go. Instead of this we know what happened and what is happening now.

Against this devotion to mere "opinions" Grauvogl raised his voice. He also has some pertinent remarks as to what is a "Simile." He says: "The substance of the law of similarity consists in this, that it indicates a correspondence in *form* which must be present for the purpose of a cure between "the form of the reaction against some morbid matter and the form of the reaction against some drug manifested in a proving. The law of similarity refers only to the *indication*, and the effect which follows is naturally not a similar but its direct contrary. Thus the strife of the *Contrarium* with the *Simile* is a strife about nothing—a strife about mere ideas of relation. The investigation of facts with a criticism based on natural laws has in all these controversies been consistently neglected."

Grauvogl was as true a Homœopath as ever lived, but he never mistook Homœopathy for being something which it is not, or ever worshipped the dogma as a kind of theological fetish. He was a truth-seeker always, and was able to find it everywhere—even in his own errors. "Errors are (or contain) often the germ of truth where the mind without a teacher is obliged to teach itself." Lest any should think there was any weakness in his apprehension of Homœopathic truth I will quote a passage from Part II, p. 390 :

"The doctrine of high potencies is the most glorious acquisition of Homœopathy. It developed its greatness and might in an intellect which has lit up the path of natural science for more than half a century, without, however, having been comprehended. And what are the discoveries of the spectrum analysis compared to the discovery of Hahnemann's high potencies ?

CHAPTER II

THE MORBID CONSTITUTIONS ACCORDING TO VARIOUS AUTHORS

MANY observers in all schools have noticed certain tendencies to particular disease-manifestations in certain types of individuals, and among those who have succeeded in reducing the different forms to specific types there is a fairly unanimous selection of the number THREE.

After years of patient observation Hahnemann saw that a superficial symptom-resemblance between drug-symptoms and disease-symptoms was sometimes insufficient to show the true specific correspondence. Eventually he tracked down the underlying constitutional dyscrasiæ to the three "miasms," and he named them, Syphilis, Sycosis and Psora. The first of these was due to the initial sore of the chancre, the second to the constitutional effects of gonorrhœa and the third to the chronic effects of itch poisoning. The three typical remedies indicated in the three dyscrasiæ were (1) *Mercury*, (2) *Thuja*, (3) *Sulphur*. These were the typical remedies of each of the three classes.

Bazin again reduces all chronic diseases to *three forms :* Scrofula, Gout, and Syphilis, from which he thinks that all other pathological forms originate.

Rademacher again, also found a three-fold division. His division was an ætiological or causative one, and varied as the peculiar cause at work. In some epidemics one type would rule and the remedy for that type would be *Copper*. At another season a somewhat different type would prevail and for that *Iron* would be needed; for a third again *Cubic Nitre* or *Natrum Nitricum* would be the remedy. And each of these remedies had allied remedies of its own type.

Grauvogl, who did not deny the value of these classifications, did not find that any of them went far enough or deep enough. So he re-stated them in terms of the tissues themselves. He also widened their borders.

It was through Hahnemann's insistence on the necessity of observing *Concomitant Circumstances* in relation to symptoms that Grauvogl was led to make his great generalisation. In the practice of Homœopathy it makes all the difference whether a symptom is *worse* or *better* in hot weather or cold, wet or dry, summer or winter. Grauvogl with his critical and analytical instincts asked himself what these conditions meant in the organism. Being well versed in chemistry, he asked himself what changes in the organism took place differently under these different conditions and he tracked them down in the first place to the changes that take place in the blood in respiration.

The animal body, solid as it looks, is made up in two thirds of its bulk of water. "It (water) is used for keeping up the physical properties of the body, and renders function and nutrition possible. It is a universal solvent chemically employed for dissolving solid substances and mechanically as a carrier of the insoluble. Water is lacking in no part of the organism and it is in relation to the manifold solid matters its most universal unit. The whole nutrition consists in the new formation of *hydrates* for supplying the place of that which is dissolved and excreted, and forms by that alone an immense *source of heat*; the water of the body absorbs *all kinds of gases* and thus alone respiration and access of oxygen becomes possible. Every process of combustion is preceded by a *polarisation of oxygen.* Ozone vanishes in the combinations which arise as products of combustion; the antozone (positively electrified ozone) remains with the water for which it has an affinity. The water can also supply the place of acids and bases, and is amphoter (both), and with a mixed food oxygen is expired, which is followed at the expense of the oxygen contained in the carbohydrates, while with the exhaled hydrogen a small quantity of *peroxide of hydrogen* is mixed. Water maintains the equilibrium of the normal temperature of the organism, while neither the blood nor the nerve centres alone regulate the production of heat." (I. p. 116.)

Respiration is a function which is not confined to the lungs, all parts of the body respire and consequently oxygen is found in all organs and tissues, sometimes as ozone (neutral) and sometimes as antozone (positive). The air we breathe is composed of Oxygen, Carbon, Hydrogen and Nitrogen, of which the whole organism is composed and which are even contained free in the blood. Thus changes of the atmospheric constituents affect the constant whole of the organism.

It is in this conception as explaining Hahnemann's observation of the effect of the various seasons and climatic conditions on patients and drug-provers that Grauvogl's arrangement of the Constitutions is based. "The Homœopath *abstracts* first from the symptoms the individuality of the patients in connection with the state of the outer world in which they have existed from their birth and out of which the *bodily constitution* is developed. The *bodily constitution* is hence the *general* cause."

Grauvogl made the true observation that if the organism is not able to adapt itself to varying conditions there is something wrong with the organism. "If, for example, a patient with intermittent fever, even before his sickness, was always affected by damp weather, *he is not cured*, even though the last paroxysm occurred years ago, *so long as he does not feel quite as well in damp as in dry weather*.

"Or, if a patient who has been for a long time annoyed by this circumstance that *every draught of air* affects him unpleasantly, *he is not cured*, even if, for instance, many years have elapsed since he recovered from his last pneumonia. As long as the disposition to take cold is not removed from him, every relapse to which he is exposed under such circumstances is proof of the *still present conditions* for the same or a similar disease, and hence a proof that *he is not wholly cured.*

"Such constitutional conditions which make themselves known by such accompanying circumstances, give us, hence, the only right indications."

No further elaboration is needed in order to show how the mind of von Grauvogl worked to map out the "generals" and to find the basic remedies for the constitutions out of which arose such a multiplicity of apparently different diseases but really only different manifestations of one and the same disease.

As a sample of that I may refer to Case IX, p. 57, in which he treated by correspondence a well-known colleague of his own, and I should like to ask any strict Hahnemannian if he thinks that even Dr. Kent himself could have found the simillimum for that plethora of symptoms.

Before passing on to a consideration of the three constitutions themselves there are one or two pregnant passages which it is well to put on record here.

"*Every living organism moves within oscillatory rhythm within various spaces of time from one position of equipoise to another.* We see this in the rhythm of the motions of our solar system even, and in its influence excited through the movements of the moon and the earth upon ourselves. But no oscillatory rhythm of life remains the same; it never returns again to the point which it last reached." (§ 200.)

I have put on the title page a sentence from Paracelsus which might have been used as a text for the following:

"To understand a disease or a cure is utterly impossible if one does not know the *history* of its development. But where is the *historic* knowledge with regard to Pathology and Therapeutics which possesses the key to these histories of development? No Clinic speaks thereof. The lectures of the Professors are silent." (§290.)

"Acute diseases run their course so to say in the track marked out by the bodily constitutions." (§ 291.)

Chapter III

THE THREE CONSTITUTIONS OF GRAUVOGL

We are now in a position to approach definitely Grauvogl's own arrangement of the morbid constitutions according to excess or deficiency of certain elements in the tissues and blood. For *every organ and every tissue breathes*, and if the lungs are the gate-way and the blood the carrier it is the tissues which are the ultimate recipients of the oxygen that is inbreathed.

1. The Hydrogenoid Constitution is characterised by an excess of Hydrogen and consequently of water in the blood and tissues.

2. The Oxygenoid is characterised by an excess of Oxygen, or, at least, by an exaggerated influence of Oxygen on the organism.

3. The Carbo-nitrogenoid Constitution is characterised by an excess of Carbon and Nitrogen.

The Hydrogenoid Constitution corresponds closely with Hahnemann's Sycosis but it covers a much wider area and is not by any means confined to the acquired or inherited results of gonorrhœal infection. Intermittent-fevers and periodicity come within its sphere.

At the present time Vaccinosis, or the constitutional sufferings from cow-pox infection, should certainly be included under this heading.

The antidotal relation to it of *Thuja*, which is one of Grauvogl's principal remedies for Hydrogenoids is a clear indication that this is so. Moreover, Burnett told me that he regarded Gout as belonging to the Sycotic diseases.

The Oxygenoid Constitution corresponds to Hahnemann's Syphilis but we have no examples of its treatment as we have of the other two.

The Carbo-nitrogenoid Constitution is Hahnemann's Psora.

I will now let Grauvogl describe them in detail and give examples of their treatment—at least of the first and third. The Hydrogenoid is the one most fully elaborated and illustrated by a great wealth of clinical cases. It is also illustrated by cases from other writers, making altogether as fascinating a clinical record as it has ever been my lot to peruse. Parts of it had been already familiar to me but I may here confess that this is the first time I have ever had an opportunity of putting the experiences in their proper setting. I trust it may prove a worthy one and as helpful to others as it has been to myself.

Chapter IV

THE HYDROGENOID CONSTITUTION

Von Grauvogl shall now speak for himself:

"This much has become clear at any rate from the investigations which have been made, that there is a constitution of the body which in many cases is the product of gonorrhœal contagion. But one would greatly err, as already said, in concluding therefrom that in this matter the question were *only* as to the consequences of a sycotic contagion. For the cause of those diseases which Hahnemann arranged under the head of Sycosis is not the only cause of the development of this state of the body which is distinguished by *a too great* proportion of water, or by hygroscopic blood.

"I always recognise this constitution of the body by the *circumstances accompanying* any disease whatever, and for which I always inquire as soon as the patient has told his complaints.

"If the patient states that he feels *worse* in cold, or damp weather, and in the rain, then I know that I have to choose among the remedies which are similar to his disease, such only as contain a greater percentage of a combination of O with C and H, consequently produce more heat and diminish the influence of the water. Hence the symptoms of a disease in this constitution of the body are *aggravated* by everything which in any way increases the atoms of water in the organism, by baths, for example, and that all the same whether they are mineral baths or simple water baths; or whatever increases the attractions of the organic molecules for water, as, for example, the eating of animals which have lived in the water, as fishes, etc. All diseases in such constitutions are *increased* by cold, also by cold and cooling food and drinks, for example, sour milk, hard eggs, cucumbers and mushrooms, but chiefly by living near water, and especially standing water.

"This experience is to me of all the more inestimable worth since I have quite cured many, very many patients simply and solely on this ground, who have been sent for years by other physicians from one bath to another, where they never found any relief and often the most marked exacerbation of their sufferings.

"Another sign that a disease has occurred in such a bodily constitution I find in the *periodicity* of its phenomena, and chiefly in its *irregular and paroxysmal* course. For even the nervous system which, next to the brain in proportion to the other parts of the body, possesses by far the greatest percentage of *water* reacts on a plus of water with an energy commensurate with that with which it carries over its reflex influence on the blood and other organic formations. The experiences of Rademacher and Hahnemann agree with this also, and these, naturally, should stand much higher in the regard of practising physicians than the researches of experimental physiology. I do not mean by this merely the one, two, three, four or eight day exacerbations and remissions, but even those periods during which for a still longer time no disease seems to exist, and this extends even over months.

"Hence for the sake of brevity I distinguish this constitution of the body, according to its *causes and conditions*, as the *Hydrogenoid*.

"I wish also to call attention to the effect of the electricity of the earth, for those nervous affections which are exacerbated by electric disturbances appear under this bodily constitution.

"In cases where there is a combination of the hydrogenoid and carbo-nitrogenoid constitutions the Hydrogenoid must be cured first and then the Carbo-nitrogenoid. This corresponds with Hahnemann's directions regarding Sycosis and Psora—Sycosis was to be dealt with first. [The same applies to Vaccinosis. —J.H.C.]

"In regard to the *Remedies* for this constitution, those substances must be curative of it which prevent the influence of the water on the blood, and here above all others I reckon *Glauber's Salts* —*Natrum sulph.* The correct indications escaped Radcmacher's adherents only because they will not use a "fool's dose" as they name the Homœopathic dilutions, whilst in their doses, that is the purgative doses, *Glauber's Salts* cannot manifest that effect.

"Since in this constitution in which Hydrogen frequently seems to have usurped the place of Nitrogen the problem is not only to diminish the influence of the Hydrogen but, where it is possible, to preserve at the same time tissues rich in nitrogen, *Nat. sul.* recommends itself all the more as Prof. Seegen has given experimental proof that by its action the exchange of the nitrogenous tissue-elements is considerably curtailed, the animal body becomes richer in nitrogenous atoms, gelatine and albuminous bodies, and that during the use of *Nat. sul.* the elements of the body free from nitrogen, and especially the fatty tissues, are more freely exchanged.

"If we know, further, that the alkalis essentially promote the operation of oxygen by means of the respiratory process, it is clear that if we compare the various localisations of the pathological processes in these constitutions and their specific forms with the Homœopathic drug-provings, then even *Nat. nitric.*, *Nat. carb.*, *Nat. acet.*, and *Sal ammoniac* (Ammonia muriatica) especially belong here.

"Moreover, in this series we may mention as nutrition remedies—[Grauvogl divides remedies into *functional* and *nutritional*]—*Calc. carb.*, *Mag. carb.*, *Mag. phos.*, and *Silica*.

"Then for other reasons adduced, *Iodine*, *Bromine*, *Chlorine*, *Nitr. ac.*, *Borax*, *Antimony*, *Alumen*, *Thuja*, *Carb. veg.*, *Arnica*, *Aranea diadema*, *Pulsatilla*, *Nux vomica* in alternation with *Ipec.*, or with *Arsen.*, *Conium*, *Apis*, *Spigelia* and animal food." (§ 308.)

In his comments on the last of the Hydrogenoid cases reported by him Grauvogl has some pertinent remarks on *Alternations* and some further remarks on *Nat. sul.* which I will quote (II. p. 374):

"Here is another practical proof that the dictum to give under no circumstances more than one remedy at a time is not always applicable.

"Since our Materia Medica contains, as yet, nothing of this effect of *Nat. sulph.* (though as a remedy it is indispensable) I have at the same time given another example that we may greatly expand and complete the Materia Medica as well as the other doctrines of Homœopathy by means of *induction.*

"If, for instance, the provings of substances of the outer world on man produce symptoms of disease which are similar to those which arise from the unintentional introduction of morbid matter, then these establish the well-known indications according to the law of similars.

"But, by this law, however, we are not taught anything regarding these various molecular substances themselves and the relation of these molecular substances and their effects on each other, and on the reaction of the organism. The two are in entirely different domains of science —of mind and of matter. These relations can be investigated and explained only according to the chemico-physical laws within the organism.

"We can explore the chemico-physical motions and counter-motions which remedies produce in the organism only by *induction*, and when we have learned thereby that *Nat. sulph.* diminishes the influence of Hydrogen on the blood, we can only come to the conclusion that the symptoms of *Nat. sulph.* must be similar to those morbid symptoms which it can cure." (II. 375.)

He goes on to say that the symptoms removed by *Nat. sulph.* should be added to the Materia Medica, which thus can be greatly enriched. This is a dictum which I can confirm from experience, and which justifies the incorporation of symptoms observed to disappear under a remedy—clinical symptoms or cured symptoms—as well as symptoms from direct provings.

CHAPTER V

EXAMPLES OF THE HYDROGENOID CONSTITUTION FROM GRAUVOGL'S PRACTICE*

CASE I.

Catalepsy, etc.—Nux. and Ipec. *in alternation ; later* Aranea diadema.

A woman, 29, of healthy parents still living (the father 89, mother 75), has suffered from her youth according to her statement, on the slightest bodily exertion or mental emotion from palpitation of the heart. The only cause she could think of was that in her youth she was very timid and easily frightened, which she ascribed to hearing children's tales. Physical examination revealed neither valvular nor other defects except rapid action even during complete bodily rest ; the pulse was 80.

Of children's diseases she had had whooping-cough and nothing else. The colour of her skin is brilliant white, the skin clear, having never presented any eruptions, hair dark-brown, eyes blue, figure slender, form symmetrical. She had already given birth to three children without difficulty, but has suffered with an incessant headache since her last confinement, which was quite normal, and after

* The cases are given in v. Grauvogl's own words.

which she nursed her child for two months, when she weaned it for lack of milk. All this happened six years before she came to see me. The headache occupied no definite place but extended from the forehead over to the occiput, only sometimes it was most severe on the vertex. This headache did not permit her to visit or receive visits from her most intimate friends even, because it was so greatly < by talking or hearing others talk that vomiting ensued; and to make the pain at all endurable she had to take to her bed, where she remained three or four days motionless and lying on her back.

Not unfrequently pain in the stomach set in which ceased of itself after the discharge of sour water rising in the throat with nausea, and also the eructations of tasteless gas, which was more frequently induced by the ingestion of vegetable acids or vegetables. Her appetite was good but not ravenous; she refused to eat meat, even the smell of it was repugnant to her. The menses, as indeed was indicated by the pain in the vertex, were irregular, scanty and pale, and were generally six to eight days too early. In the interval there was more or less leucorrhœa which was debiliting, and the accession of the menses was announced by a violent colic.

The respiration was unrestrained, but in the apex of the right lung there was a dull respiratory murmur, in a small portion without any change of sound on percussion. She never had any cough and the digestion was regular.

To the above symptoms were added, since her last confinement also, *cataleptic attacks*, almost every morning, after waking from an uninterrupted, good, but not refreshing sleep. Thus, if her husband did not notice in the morning that she closed her eyes again shortly after waking, and at the same time sighed once deeply, and at this very moment did not at once shake her shoulders with both hands and call to her aloud, then nothing would arouse her from the motionless insensible condition lasting from one to two hours, in which one could raise her arms and legs in any direction without them returning to their former position. These attacks had come and still came and went without any known cause, but they left behind them no further ailment.

As regards the *concomitant circumstances* of these pains, I learned that they were much more violent *in damp weather* than in dry and, in fact, her general condition was < at such times, so that this woman, who was previously lively and joyful became more and more melancholic. The many physicians who had been consulted, the many cures which had been tried for her, and especially *all use of baths*, increased her sufferings. I further learned that her headache especially, even aside from considering the influence of the weather, was most violent in the afternoon and evening; that consequently it increased in severity irregularly though *periodically*, which also pointed to an affection of the nervous system; that she constantly suffered from *chilliness*, hence the whole winter through was obliged to keep her room very warm, and even in summer she had *cold hands* and feet, notwithstanding all her clothing and other means for keeping warm.

Whoever has read the foregoing will have no doubt that here we have before us a disease in a *hydrogenoid* constitution, which latter must be extirpated first of all, without regard to the organs affected or the other parts of the organism ; for as long as the *general* conditions of a disease are not removed no thought can ever be logically entertained of the cure or improvement of its *special* form.

I often read in the Homœopathic journals clinical cases of physicians whose treatment, contravening this logical principle, was followed by little good results, or less than that which really was obtainable ; while, by virtue of the Law of Similarity other physicians again were led to the right indication, though this principle was unknown to them. This is, then, an involuntary logic of the Homœopaths, as a counterpart to the involuntary Homœopathy of the physiological school.

I know full well that, unhappily, few Homœopathists trouble themselves about the physiological significance of remedies, but in the choice of these remedies they are all the more uncertain inasmuch as our drug-provings still require complements.

In brief, among all the remedies which might be indicated according to the law of similarity for the case, which certainly was not easily to be cured, there were mainly two of which I knew at once from many years practice, that they not only produce a more active interchange of substance, and hence would occasion more warmth in the body, and would not only restore the lost power of resistance against the influences of cold and moisture, but would also have an enlivening effect on the nervous system. These two are *Nux vomica* and *Ipecac.* I have also observed that each of these remedies had far less effect in these directions when given by itself, alone, than when they were permitted to operate on the organism in succession.

I therefore ordered *Nux* 3 to be taken at 7 or 8 a.m. and 6 p.m., and three or four drops of *Ipec.* 3, every two hours during the day, although it was the fervent desire of this patient to be delivered as soon as possible, first of all and at any price, from the headache which tormented her without ceasing, for this was the most annoying of all her sufferings and hindered her in most of her duties.

Had I sought to conform to this wish I should surely have had to select quite other remedies, and probably a long series of them in succession, and most probably too with no favourable result —or no result at all.

Hence I told the patient that I could not meet her wishes at once but on the other hand promised her with all assurance the complete restoration of her health and, within the space of a year at furthest, a deliverance from all her sufferings; adding that before her headache could be relieved she would first have to notice a greater sensation of warmth in her body.

Besides, I forbade her to take any baths for more than five minutes, and for the time being her accustomed washing in cold water; and also her remaining near water, especially standing water. I forbade her also coffee and, of course, vinegar, fruit and fish.

This was on the 1st of May. I visited the patient every eight days, having told her to take the remedies as directed for eight days, and then to set them aside for eight days, and so on.

On the 4th of June she stated that she really thought she was not so cold as she had been for many years, for she could now even sit in the shade in the garden, a thing which had hitherto been impossible to her. At the same time the cataleptic attacks had so diminished in intensity that she had often only a mere intimation of them. But headache and palpitation of the heart still unfitted her for all occupation.

The cataleptic attacks now happily had returned but seldom for several weeks (except the merest indication of them), and even the headaches were no longer aggravated in the evening, when, at the end of July, her children got measles one after the other. She would not entrust the care of them to anybody but was unspeakably happy that she could sustain the bodily exertions and mental excitements thereupon attendant, which a month before would have been utterly impracticable.

During the whole course of her children's sickness I naturally intermitted the use of the *Ipecac.* and *Nux*, and only gave her *Aconite* occasionally, as she was very much alarmed at the condition of one of the children whose disease had become very severe.

After this had all passed off without injury for the children as well as for the mother, the whole family went for eight days into the mountains of Bavaria. This agreed very well with all except the mother; for she *took a sail upon a lake*, which I had expressly forbidden, and after this day felt chilly and cold again, the headache also being notably aggravated.

As I had found in my practice that *Aranea diadema* even more than *Nux.* and *Ipec.* diminishes the influence of hydrogen upon the system, and since it was also indicated according to the law of similars, I directed her to take four or five drops every two hours.

The warmth of the body soon returned, and for the first time the menses waited for the full four weeks, but was more abundant and of a red colour. It is a pity that in other cases, the *Aranea diadema* produces very violent hæmorrhage, especially from the lungs, which fact calls for caution in the use of this great remedy.

After two weeks the patient noticed a marked relief of the headaches which had returned; and after eight days this headache entirely ceased for some days. The cataleptic attacks had already entirely disappeared for about a fortnight and have not returned since. But it was not till the 13th of September that the patient finally assured me that, in the most striking manner, just as if she had been delivered from a bad habit, she had not had the slightest sensation of a headache for four days.

Nor has it ever returned again after the lapse of six years.

After another fortnight, during which time the patient had personally superintended the removal from her summer residence to the city, a thing which before was not to be thought of, she called my attention to the fact that after having been in the city three days she had experienced increased palpitation of the heart again, as had been the case every year after this change. Now I gave her *Puls.* 30, since the constitutional conditions for the previous ailments were all removed. As the favourable effects of the 30th began to wear off in a few days I gave *Puls.* 3. This had the desired effect within six days and the heart's action became regular and remained so.

I now gave her finally *Magnes. sulph.* 6, after which even her leucorrhœa diminished, and now disappeared entirely, not to return.

Thus, at the end of November of this year this woman was perfectly free from all her sufferings of years' standing. She went into society again and renewed her youth.

From the above rule and a large experience I know that neither *Puls.* nor *Magnes. sulph.* would have afforded relief so readily had not the constitutional treatment preceded.

NOTE ON *Aranea diadema.*

In addition to the already known symptoms of *Aranea* and the above quoted symptoms as regards hæmorrhages, the following have been obtained from a proving on a healthy woman :

At night, immediately after lying down,

sudden violent pains in the teeth of the upper and lower jaw.

Periods eight days too early, too strong and too copious.

Numbness and formication of ring and little fingers of both hands.

Case II.

Hydrogenoid Intermittent. Aranea diadema.

A pupil of the Academy of Arts, 23, sent for me because he could no longer pursue his art with love and pleasure; he felt himself so constantly oppressed in the chest that a walk across the room even put him out of breath. He attributed his troublo to an *intermittent fever* acquired in a university city some months before, which was removed by very large doses of *Quinine*, of which he often had to take 20 grains at once. Since that time *an enlargement of the spleen* had remained which reached to the space between third and fourth ribs. At that place a dark line made on the skin with Nitrate of Silver by the professor of the City Hospital to mark the outlines of the enormous swelling of the spleen was still visible. Below the first line there were other reddish marks, the traces of similar outlines which had indicated the gradual swelling and ascent of the spleen. The heart was pushed to the right and beat feebly, 98 to tho minute. The respiration was very short, raised the right side of the thorax only, 30 times to the minute, and audible only at the very apex of the right lung.

The appearance of this young man of course indicated disease of the spleen. The upper edge was found again between the third and fourth ribs, though in consequence of earlier improvement, it must previously have stood lower.

As soon as I entered the house where he resided and which stood *close to the water*, I observed that all the walls were very damp. I was now convinced that I should find a disease-form arising from a hydrogenoid constitution, for such a house, especially when it is but little or not at all exposed to the sun, is very sure to harbour disease-forms of the most varied kinds, but which ought not to be treated according to their names as they are set down in the text-books of special Pathology and Therapeutics in which their treatment is struck off after one and the same model.

Here, however, the disease was a relapse induced by the damp dwelling. On being questioned the patient said that *he was chilly* day and night, although it was midsummer, and *as often as it rained* he had always felt worse. He also acknowledged that especially during the past four weeks, during which time he had lived in this room, he had felt worse than ever.

On constitutional grounds, as well as on the strength of the indication of the law of similars, there was no doubt that the remedy indicated was *Aranea diadema*. He was ordered it in the 2*x*, four or five drops in a spoonful of water every two hours.

After eight days the upper border of the spleen was behind the fifth rib and fell within six weeks to the seventh. The heart returned to its place ; and in the part of the lung which had been compressed the respiratory murmur was again distinctly heard, and the patient felt himself well again. Nevertheless I advised him to continue the remedy some time longer. Some days after, however, he complained of acute pains in the teeth of the upper and lower jaws which had occurred for two days when he retired at night and lasted an hour.

In this case it was a fortunate chance that I had already learned this symptom of *Aranea* from provings. Yet this case serves again as an example of the diagnosis of the so-called Homœopathic aggravation ; of a diagnosis which is always justified on the basis of drug-provings. Not a single adherent of the physiological school possesses that acquaintance with the effects of his remedies which could explain to him similar aggravations. Even this important condition for the frequent elimination of the accidental at the sick-bed is utterly unknown to the physiological school and is one of the causes of a host of mistakes.

The physiological school has collected some very valuable facts regarding the relations of the water in the atmosphere to that of the organism, but it does not know of what good they might be for its Therapy, for it lacks the knowledge of how to find remedies against diseases arising from a surplus of hydrogen in the organism. Thus Hemming in his " Doctrine of the Causes of Disease " says :

" The lungs exhale an air saturated with

hydrogen gas of a temperature of 37½°C., 30° R. [99.4°F.]. If the surrounding air, at a temperature of 37½°C. were saturated with hydrogen gas, then as much hydrogen gas would be offered to the organism through the lungs as is given off. But since this is not the case the blood in the lungs gives off to the dry atmosphere determinate quantities of water.

"Still greater is the interchange through the skin and the excretion of water by the kidneys. The exhalation of water through the lungs amounts on the average in 24 hours to 354 grammes; by the skin to 720; and through the kidneys to 1,369.3 grammes.

"The mean proportion of water in the healthy organism is 79 per cent, while there are large numbers of individuals whose blood contains more water and others whose blood is richer in solid constituents. The cause of Chlorosis is scanty exerction of water from the organism, together with a mode of living which allows of the formation of few solid constituents in the blood. The scanty excretion of water is caused by living in an air relatively damp, by too little bodily exercise and by deficient expansion of the lungs.

"The swelling of the spleen has developed before the outbreak of the intermittent and is the cause and not the effect of the febrile attacks; the enormous perspiration produced by the paroxysm is the attempt of nature to remove the fundamental cause of the watery character of the blood and the swelling of the spongy body of the spleen therefrom arising."

All the above are very good indications for practice, which Homœopaths alone know how to make use of. Could Flemming have found the remedy for this case? Certainly not, since the Physiological Materia Medica makes no mention of *Aranea diadema*.

[Commenting on the above case Dr. Jousset remarked that the "swollen spleen" was possibly a big pleuritic effusion. But this makes no difference to the fact of the Hydrogenic cure.]

Case III.

Sycotic Neuralgia. Natrum sulph.

For many years I have known a vigorous young man of herculean musculature and form, with most blooming countenance and cheerful temper. After a few years I saw him, quite as powerful as ever, it is true, but labouring now under *mental depression.* As I fear nothing so much as to appear obtrusive, I could not ask him any further questions, especially as he had assured me in reply to the usual enquiries that he was very well. A few years later again he came to consult me about certain attacks which alarmed him very much although he had already consulted on this account several of the most eminent physicians and had received from them the same assurance that these attacks had all the less importance *as they always disappeared of themselves very rapidly and completely*, in short, that they were no objects of medical treatment.

The sum and substance of the whole complaint was, indeed, trifling enough to the ignorant, and was as follows: "Within a period of three years it has already happened to me three times when in perfect health, and the last time three days ago, that when walking I am *suddenly taken with such an acute stitch* in the left hip as utterly disables me from walking further because it is absolutely impossible to stand on that foot since it becomes so weakened as to be utterly incapable of furnishing any support. This stitching pain is so severe that *I think for the moment that I shall lose my senses* and must fall to the ground every moment; that I am sure I could not bear it if it lasted but a minute; the pain of having a tooth drawn being child's play compared to it, and no words can describe it. But the strangest thing is that, in the very moment when it seems as if I must succumb to it, *it disappears without leaving a trace just as suddenly, and apparently just as much without cause, as it came*, after having lasted according to my calculation two or three seconds, and I can at once go on my way as if nothing had happened. Before and after it I am quite well; but the dread of never being secure for a moment against this most fearful of all pains does not allow me to rest till I find help, and indeed I am all the more disquieted by it as the last time the pain was not only in the hip but at the same time reached to the knee joint."

This symptom was already known to me as a precursor of sycosis in a high state of development, and although the patient assured me that he had always been quite well, I had him undress himself and found upon his chest the characteristic exanthem which he made very light of, since now it mostly broke out in the Spring, now soon disappeared of itself, while during the *whole Summer and Winter it was not to be seen*, and he thought it was to be attributed to the time of year. On further enquiry I learned that three years ago a friend of his, a physician, had touched some *whitish-blue spots*, which he showed him *on his lips* with *Nitrate of Silver*, whereupon after a few days they disappeared and have never re-appeared since. Moreover, he was often overtaken with such a disgust for life that he had to summon all his moral force to refrain from shooting himself, though he did not know any other cause for this than a disheartening disgust for life. Beyond this I could learn nothing, and as regards any results from sexual intercourse, he assured me that he had never observed any whatever. We know very well how little we can credit such statements. In the meantime it was not essential to know whether such a cause had existed or not, for a pathological form is always the *combined result* of causes and conditions ; hence the specific disease-form according to time, place and circumstance, is *the only object of Therapeutics*. For the sake of curiosity I examined a drop of his blood, which contained, however, no more colourless corpuscles than is customary in non-leucœmic blood.

It had long been known to me that at the outset of the so-called Sycotic cases *the percentage of water of the blood is increased*, as also in the later stages, in which Virchow had discovered leucœmic blood. It was also known to me that Glauber's Salts protected the red corpuscles from the influence of an excess of water, while in Brüminghausen, Handschuk, Wilhelm, Klurge, etc., I had men before me of great powers of observation, who were in favour of treating syphilis with Glauber's Salts, but who are long ago forgotten, because Sycosis and Syphilis were confounded and there was no indication for Glauber's Salts in the latter disease and as a matter of fact it never accomplished anything. Thus both theoretical and practical experience sustained me, which left no doubt in me that Glauber's Salts were indicated for this case. I did not acquire certainty, however, except through the Homœopathic provings of Glauber's Salts—*Natrum sulphuricum*—likewise known to me in so far as this that no other remedy belonging to this category presents these relations to the hip and knee joints in connection with other circumstances as do Glauber's Salts. Without hesitation I prescribed *Nat. sul.* 3*x*, five drops every two hours. Since prescriptions which are based not only on theoretical and practical experience, but also on the law of specific direction, or the law of similars, can never fail of success, so did the result not fail in this case, although it required nearly a year to complete, and to guard against supersaturating the system the remedy was often set aside for weeks together. After this period, however, there was no trace of the exanthem to be seen, the former cheerfulness of the patient as well as his blooming complexion had returned, and since he has now passed five years in this desirable condition without further use of the remedy and without complaints, I may consider the cure to be complete.

Case IV.

Latent Intermittent Simulating Consumption. Chinin. sulph.

A married woman, 29, suffered from a cough for eight years without any known cause, the cough having every year terminated in pulmonary hæmorrhage. Four years ago she had for six months pains in the face on the right side, which would yield to no medical means of the physiological school, though these pains ceased of themselves after a change of residence ; hereupon, however, the cough, *which during the continuance of the pains had disappeared, returned again*, so that the woman became much emaciated, and had to drink Ems water at her own house since, on account of her weakness she could not be taken to Ems. By this means, however, her strength was so far restored that the following year she was able herself to go to Ems there to continue the cure.

After four weeks *she returned home no better.* Blood was always present in the copious puriform expectoration, and her physician, who only saw her every week or two, told her husband that his wife was incurable. She herself, believing what the physician said of her hopeless condition, became *despondent*, and her condition sensibly grew worse.

She now thought of consulting me. Her husband requested me, after telling me everything, and after all hope of any improvement had long been given up, at least to pay her a visit.

One cannot refuse even such a somewhat unreasonable demand. I found a woman in a great state of depression, always weeping, with marked mucous rattle on the right upper part of the chest, and on the left side as well as the right a clear sound on percussion, puriform expectoration, constant irritation to cough under the sternum. *The menses, however, were not yet deranged, appetite and sleep were good, pulse 72 ; the face was very pale but did not have the expression of the tuberculous.* On being questioned she assured me that she had long ago observed that she had *two good days and one poor one, and that only in damp weather did she suffer all days alike ;* that she had told this to her physician many years before, but he had always said that it was irrelevant, as well as the circumstance that she always had *cold feet and hands.*

I could now no longer doubt that here a latent intermittent had existed for eight years, and the remedy which I gave, *Chinin. sulph.*, a dose every two hours, had such an effect that, from the first day the cough became less frequent and on the eighth day had entirely disappeared. The patient soon appeared very happy and gained in strength from day to day.

Since then four years have elapsed and there has never been any return of the cough, or of the hæmorrhage, and the abnormalities on the upper part of the lungs could no longer be observed.

This woman, granting that I saved her life, would have been buried long since as surely as the treatment of her physician of the physiological school was a false one; because these physicians, on account of the knowledge which they have obtained mechanically, and of which they always boast as infallible, are not able in such cases to establish a true diagnosis; for they cannot, and never could, estimate the circumstances accompanying any disease-form.

Case V.

Uterine Fibroma in a Hydrogenoid. Nux and Ipec.

A married woman, 28, who gave birth to her last child some years ago without difficulty, and who appeared to have no predisposition to any disease, complained that for six months her abdomen had been greatly enlarging to such an extent that everyone had been congratulating her on a new pregnancy, which, however, could not be the case, as she had none of the usual indications. Her periods were regular, every four weeks as usual and only for a few weeks she had had a constant leucorrhœa. The abdomen was round and everywhere uniformly hard all round in a circumference of about six inches diameter above the symphysis pubis, but it was entirely free from pain even on pressure. An examination showed a condition of the os uteri as in the fourth month of pregnancy. The os was high and directed backwards.

Around it, in the bottom of the vagina, the same cartilaginous resistance was felt as externally on the abdomen, and this resistance formed the immediate prolongation of the cervix and thus belonged to the womb. I have twice happened to observe a similar swelling of the womb arising from a dead fœtus ; in one case the fœtus lay five and in the other eleven months in the uterine cavity without being expelled. In the first case metritis suddenly set in and during its course, which could not be mitigated, the separate bones of the fœtus were discharged one after the other through the rectum. The other case escaped my further observation. Both cases were free from doubt by means of the signs of pregnancy which had been manifestly present, and in the latter case even the parts of the fœtus could be distinctly felt. All this was absent here. Thus it could only be considered a fibrous polypus, or, more probably, a round fibroid within the uterus.

Owing to the size of the growth an operation was not to be thought of, though to the physiological school any other resource is unknown. Consequently this woman would have been given over hopelessly, a prey to all the dangers which were to be anticipated in the case.

What may deliver us from such a dilemma ? Nothing but the teaching of Homœopathy touching the *Concomitant Circumstances.*

This woman *did not look at all ill, had a good appetite and slept well, only she became sooner more wearied by her domestic duties than was previously the case,* in the discharge of which duties she was very much incommoded by this tumour in her abdomen.

This was on April 4th. The remedies which I administered internally so long as I had my eye on the object of the disease alone were attended with no success, and from month to month the abdomen increased in size until—unhappily it was not till September 6th—I enquired about the concomitant circumstances. She acknowledged that she *felt chilly every evening, and was worse, that is, there was more rapid enlargement of the abdomen, during moist weather.* On this account I prescribed *Nux* 3 and *Ipec.* 3 in alternation every two hours, and with such effect that as early as September 26th the tumour had decreased in size to a diameter of three inches, though it could still be distinctly felt above the pubic bone. The cervix had also assumed a convex position and by the 30th of October had become quite perpendicular again ; the lips were somewhat swollen, but the leucorrhœa had disappeared.

The improvement continued without interruption, during frequent suspension of the remedies, and four years have passed without any complaint from the woman, so that her complete cure was certainly accomplished.

Case VI.

Hydrogenous Pneumonia. Nux *and* Ipec.; Nux *and* Aranea.

A butcher and tavern keeper, 25, was taken, according to the declaration of his physician, with so violent a pneumonia that there was no hope of his recovery. The patient, however, was about to be married and the business would have been lost to his betrothed by his death. The physician therefore advised the patient to consummate his marriage as soon as possible. This took place; but now I was called to take charge of the case, a request which, of course, I thought I had a perfect right to decline. Yet I could not withstand their repeated urgent appeals for more than a day. I found hepatisation of the whole right lung from the lowest part to the apex, above the clavicle, the sound on percussion was somewhat hollow, and there was some respiratory murmur yet to be heard. The left lung had remained free from any affection. There was great difficulty of respiration, excessive debility, voice harsh, inability to lie on the left side without danger of suffocation, pulse 130. The cough brought up purulent yet scanty expectoration, the tongue was thickly coated, appetite entirely wanting. There was great emaciation with collapsed features.

On enquiry the patient stated that *one day he was better—on the next decidedly worse, and then at 8 p.m. he was worse than ever,* so that he really thought the evening before that his time had come; he *felt chilly* also, notwithstanding the constant sweat, and in spite of the warm clothing on his abdomen. I prescribed *Nux vom.* and *Ipec.* in alternation every two hours. On the next day, August 2nd, there was amelioration of all the symptoms. After eight days he still was *chilly in the upper part of his body* hence *Aran. diadem.* 3 was given in hourly alternation with *Nux*, although the hepatisation was decreasing from above downwards more and more every day. On August 29th he was already able to remain two hours out of bed, for his appetite had returned in the first days of my treatment, and hearty food was given as his strength increased. He now felt quite well. The whole right lung was again serviceable for respiration, and in the same proportion the burden of the other ailment was also removed. The bodily weakness, however, was still considerable.

That day the young wife of the patient was standing at the door of her house as her previous physician passed by. He stopped to enquire about her husband, when, with a joyful countenance, she replied that he was quite well and already up. To this the doctor replied, "That is utterly impossible." A week later the patient himself met the doctor and gave him ocular demonstration of that which he had declared to be utterly impossible!

Case VII.

Caries of Os Calcis; Gangrenous Ulcer. Arsen., *Aggravation by* Calc. *and* Silic., *Cure by* Aranea diadema.

After opening an abscess on the left heel of a man, 75, the edges of the wound mortified and the physician declared that as *gangrena senilis* had set in the foot must be removed. Upon this decision I was called in. For more than a year

I had seen this old man in the street limping with his left foot, and now I saw clearly the cause thereof—a chronic inflammation of the periosteum of the os calcis, which had probably extended to the bone itself, and a gangrenous ulcer half an inch broad, causing insufferable pains and surrounded and partially covered with a gangrenous crust. *Arsen.* 10 gave prompt relief. The gangrenous crust was thrown off. The surface of the ulcer took on a healthy appearance, but after ten days did not show the least tendency to cicatrise, although the pains were decreasing. Both *Silic.* 10 and *Calc. c.* 10 aggravated all the symptoms so far as this that none of them were better, but the ulcer had increased in breadth and depth, so that the probe could now touch the denuded and carious os calcis. The patient wanted his first drops again because they had relieved his pains, which now had returned to their former severity. This was granted him in the absence of any better indication. But the sleeplessness setting in, which could be attributed only to the *Arsen.* required that this remedy should again be discontinued. His sleep now returned but the pain increased again also.

A thorough examination now led me to the source of all his troubles, to which, indeed, the striking effect of *Arsen.* had already called my attention, as this remedy was given only to arrest the mortification. On being questioned the patient acknowledged that his pains *increased and decreased periodically*, and that regularly, every other day. He added that he might have told me this long before had he supposed that any importance could have been attached to such a trifle. He had thought that quite as little importance was to be attached to the circumstance that *he was always cold*, and hence was always trying to get warm.

Aranea diadema removed the pains and affected a rapid cure. At first the ulcer grew less; then many very small sequestra were thrown off; but five months passed under the repeated use of this remedy before the cure was complete.

Hay-Baths.

I avail myself of this opportunity to call attention to the use of hay-baths in many forms of caries and in enchondroma of the bones. It was in the country that I first learned of these baths as a popular remedy for necrosis of bone. If what the country people related to me is true then it can only be the *Silex* contained in these baths which makes them useful in diseases of the bones. Hence I examined the hay chemically in order to learn whether Silex could be found in solution in these baths; and this proved to be the case.

Case VIII.

Hydrocephalus. Sulphur, Calc. phos., Arg. nit.

A young married couple had two years previously lost a child from acute hydrocephalus. The second child, then eight months old, was committed to my charge when the disease had already reached the convulsive stage, and it died in a few days.

It now devolved on me, as the family physician to solve the problem of protecting the next child from this disease and thus remove the *conditions* under which, both times, the development of this fatal disease had been possible, a problem which, as everybody knows, the physiological school is not able to solve.

Both parents were perfectly healthy and never ill. Both had blonde hair, thin skin and blue eyes. The husband was spare, the wife of full habit. Hence no positive point of support could be gained from either. The wife had nursed both children, but without having sufficient nourishment for them as I learnt on enquiry, for she was obliged to give them in addition milk and sugar-water, and both were taken ill when they began to *cut their teeth.*

In hydrocephalus the nutrition of the bones is always deficient and hence during the period of dentition this nutrition must be carried on at the expense of other tissues. But the *conditions* of this deficient nutrition of the osseous system must have given long before the period of dentition.

Hence I told the wife that she must not nurse the next child, and that she must during her next pregnancy take *Sulph.* 6 one day and *Calc. phos.* 6 the next, so that she should not lose a third child by this disease. *Sulphur* I wished to exhibit as a nutritive remedy favouring the formation of tissues, while *Calc. phos.* was to favour that of bones.

Five weeks later the woman informed me that she was again pregnant and asked me for these remedies. She was delivered at term, and this child, now five years old, remained healthy, as well as a second, now three, which was carried the regular term under this prophylactic treatment.

These are not solitary cases, for I have pursued this method for six years in all families in which there has ever been a hydroecphalie child, and with the same good result.

But where I have taken charge in other families of children who had already suffered from hydrocephalus none have died during the last seven years, during which time I have given such children every morning and evening a powder of the second trituration of *Calc. phos.*; and only such children as I first see in the last stage receive morning and evening a few drops of *Arg. nit.* 6 and every two hours the powder of *Calc. phos.* with the best result. At the same time I have repeatedly convinced myself that in such cases one of the remedies alone affords no such relief.

Case IX.

Sycosis. Thuja *and* Natrum sulph.

In September, 1861, I received from a well-known Homœopathic physician the following letter, which I give *verbatim :*

"I hope you will excuse me for taking the liberty of relating my disease to you with the request that you will kindly give me the benefit of your skill in my case.

"I am 53, of nervous constitution and have

suffered from piles since my youth. I have employed all sorts of remedies against these with but transient treatment. Subsequently a hypochondriac mood was super-added. Homœopathy and the water cure have given me but little relief from my sufferings. My manner of life from my youth up was much like that of others. I drank two or three glasses of beer every day, smoked tobacco and partook of the ordinary fare. Married at 23, I became the father of eight children, quite healthy and vigorous. I was never syphilitic, rachitic or scrofulous, but when a child was afflicted with itch which perhaps was checked too soon by means of ointments. Although I was never excessive in amorous indulgence, I always observed a pressing pain in the testicles after coitus, which was more violent as the coitus was more frequent and *vice versa*; it was < when standing but > by walking and still more on lying down. This, perhaps, may have its cause in youthful sexual sins.

"My hæmorrhoidal pains, which were especially severe in the years from 30 to 40, tormented me after every stool with their burning pains as if the parts were raw. Later in life the pain disappeared, and the hæmorrhoidal knobs were only swollen when I drank a glass of beer too much of an evening. Only very seldom was there any discharge of blood, and it was only after having used cold sitz-baths and cold injections for several years that there were repeated hæmorrhages after stool, without affording any essential relief.

"I am very nervous and hence could never take the sitz-baths under 68° Far., since if used *in a lower temperature febrile attacks were always induced.*

"In 1859 an acute burning sore pain appeared again after every stool as well as protrusion of the hæmorrhoidal tumours. The pain after stool was very severe and sometimes continued for hours. As no remedy afforded me any relief I determined to adopt a vegetarian diet. Accordingly from the beginning of September, 1859, I avoided all animal food, drank no beer, denied myself smoking and every irritant. My breakfast and supper were bread and milk; my dinner consisted of vegetables and dishes made of flour and milk; my drink was water. As a consequence I strictly resisted the greatest longing for meat. Now and then I took a dose of some Homœopathic remedy of which *Calc. carb.* and *Sepia* 200 acted most beneficially. In connection with this I practised gymnastics every day according to Dr. Neumann's directions in his 'Hausgymnastick.' My sufferings were more endurable but the hæmorrhoidal pains continued, and a melancholy as of undeserved injustice set in, with pressure in the throat, < on walking in the open air; easily wearied by a long walk causing a careless gait. Last spring I became accidentally acquainted with Braunscheidtismus and got possession of Braunscheidt's book. The great recommendations of the method against hæmorrhoids and hypochondria soon aroused a desire in me to try it. Hence I proceeded at once to carry out my plan and applied the instrument with intervals of ten days upon the back, the sacrum, the whole circumference of the abdomen, on the outer side of the thigh, on the calves seven times, and it was used the last time seven weeks ago.

The result, however, is very sad ; for after the fifth application the left axilla swelled up and became painful. Soon after I got an ulcer on the outer side of the thigh, and one on the left forearm, suppurating for a long time. Then developed a reddish knotty eruption spreading over the whole body. The tubercles of the size of a small lentil are in many places so elevated above the skin that they resembled wart-like excrescences. These have their seat chiefly on the vertex, above the ear, on the forehead, on the left side of the neck, between the scrotum and the right thigh, and scattered here and there on the penis and about the anus. Small scales form on them, they itch but little and after being scratched the itching is relieved. At the same time, above the third rib on the left side near the sternum there was a swelling, painful on pressure. My knees became stiff so that I could go upstairs only with the greatest labour. There appeared besides an oppressive weight on each shoulder, with sensitiveness thereof to pressure. Great sensitiveness in separate small portions of the thorax < by drawing a deep breath and by eructations, but soon disappearing again, now frequently annoyed me very much. The most distressing pain, however, was a rheumatic, throbbing, tearing pain in the head, which disappeared entirely, perhaps on the use of *Merc. sol.*, *Nux.* and *Byronia.* In short, after this Braunseheidtismus, as I think, a rheumatism developed itself, which has lasted now for about six weeks.

"To give a more exact detail of my case, I take the liberty of describing my present condition as follows :

"Rheumatic tensive pains on the left side of the neck. Pressing pain on the shoulders with sensitiveness of the top of the shoulders to external pressure. Pain as of dislocation in the shoulders and arms on raising the arms. Painfulness of the bones, especially of the left hand, so that I can hardly grasp and hold a small weight, a book for instance. Painfulness of the third rib on the left side on external pressure. Redness and swelling of the skin over the point of the right elbow. A slight jar with the hand upon a firm substance produced, some days ago, a dull humming pain in the hand. Painfulness of the spinous processes of two of the lumbar vertebræ on pressure (at present one only being painful). Painfulness in the right elbow joint, and on the upper part of the right arm, especially when turning the hand outwards. Paralytic weakness (and paralytic pains) of the legs, especially of the right, with painfulness of the knee-joint on extending and flexing the leg. When sitting in a chair I can raise the right leg only by keeping it extended. Raising the leg while the knee is bent is impossible on account of the pain in the knee-joint. Weakness of the knee-joint when walking in the room. Sitting down or rising from a sitting posture can only be accomplished by the most powerful support of the hands. Going up stairs is impossible. Painfulness of the heels, especially the left, when rising and afterwards, and when beginning to walk. Redness of the uvula and velum pendulum palati, with pain in the throat, especially on empty swallowing (this is much better). A red tubercular eruption about the anus and between the right thigh and the scrotum, almost like warts raised above the skin, itching but little and especially at first on the forehead, now on the forehead, now on the vertex above the ears, on the left side of the neck and on the front of the chest. Furuncles on the right arm near the axilla. For a few days past slight œdematous swelling of the feet. Respiration sighing. Pulse 90. Weeping mood; doubtful of recovery.

"I must add, however, that my pulse has always been somewhat accelerated, and that the pains seem to be seated in the bones and are < only by pressure and motion, as well as that the upper ends of the shin bones, just below the knee-joint, are painful on being pressed. Sour smelling night-sweat.

"The above symptoms have set in since the use of the Braunscheidtismus. But in order to give you a closer insight into my disease I will also give you those symptoms which have annoyed me for a long time and which are now present:

"Confusion, humming, heaviness and fulness of the head, glittering before the eyes. Roaring in the ears, mucous rattling. Heat in the mouth. Bad breath. Appetite and digestion good. Protrusion of the hæmorrhoidal tumours at stool. Burning and soreness at the anus after stool, < on walking and > by sitting and lying. Cracking of the joints ; sense of swelling and difficult motion of the fingers, < when walking in the open air and in the morning in bed. Powerlessness of the hands when writing, which is very difficult for me. Hardness and thickening of the skin on the ball of the left toe, with pains when walking on the pavement as if treading on small stones. Easy perspiration; sour-smelling perspiration. Sensation as if a fibre were torn or snapped off suddenly at the left axilla. Aching in the testicles after coitus ; > by sitting, still more by lying down. Pain in the groin from the pressure of the loins, which annoyed me very much since the Braunscheidtismus, although I have not worn the truss for fourteen days (at present relieved).

" Against this complaint I have already taken *Merc. sol.*, *Nux. vom.*, *Bryonia*, *Ant. tart.*, *Sulphur* and *Colchicum.* I have now taken *Rhus.* since September 7th. I have taken two drops of the 2x, repeated at first every six hours. Now, September 21st, I am taking a dose only morning and evening. I do not notice any striking result such as I have often seen in my practice.

" I am father of seven children yet unprovided for, without means, and the support of my large family depends entirely upon the earnings of my practice. Hence my situation at present is truly a sad one and the future looks darker still, since I fear my lower limbs may yet become paralysed."

No expert will doubt that for this disease the physiological school has no name, and since it has none it hence cannot say what is really present here, and at most could recognise as special troubles, hæmorrhoids, paralysis, etc. To establish a *Constitutional Diagnosis* is hence impossible for it, and consequently it could make neither a rational prescription nor prognosis. Neither could empiricism help in this case. Was Homœopathy as helpless as the others ?

On the contrary. After I had received this letter of September 23rd, 1861, and had reflected on it I wrote the patient as follows :

"In your letter you have given me a very good description of the phenomena which are wont to accompany the development of *Sycosis*, whether you have acquired or inherited it. Hence you will have the goodness without delay to take *Thuja* 30 morning and evening as well as *Natrum sulph.* every third hour—four or five drops of each in a spoonful of water. At the same time I beg of you not to practise great abstinence, nor to fast, for no form of sycotic disease can be cured without good food, without nutrition of the parts which remain healthy. Whether you are quite curable I would rather leave undecided at present, but in any case you can be so far restored that you will be able to resume your practice again."

Truly this strict diet, which unhappily many Homœopathists from great misunderstanding of facts insist upon even to this day, so that to a sick man actually nothing is left to live upon but the air, does by no means aid in the spread of Homœopathy, and indeed it is thus wantonly deprived of one of the greatest guarantees of its results at the bedside.

I will now give (1) the symptoms which led me to this diagnosis ; and (2) what induced me to give two remedies in alternation, an abomination to orthodox Homœopathists.

(1) The following symptoms are above all characteristic of the sycotic form of this disease : Swelling and suppuration of the axillary glands, sores on the outer side of the left leg ; tubercular wart-like eruptions on the above mentioned parts of the body ; swelling of the rib on the left side near the sternum ; stiffness of the knee, the various so-called rheumatic pains ; redness of the velum palati with painfulness of the throat on empty swallowing ; pains in the loins ; cracking of the joints ; with all the symptoms above indicated under the modern idea of the locomotor ataxy of Duchenne and Eisenmann.

(2) As regards the remarks, that according to this diagram *Thuja* is indicated needs no further discussion for those who are versed in the Homœopathic drug-provings. But *Thuja*, both according to these provings and experience at the bedside, cannot cure the tubercular, or, as our colleague expressed it, wart-like eruption ; *Natrum sulph.* alone can accomplish that. But this tubercular eruption is just the most dangerous form of this disease. If not removed at once it luxuriantly develops in many parts of the body, especially on the neck and in the region of the clavicle, and grows into great

clusters which the inexperienced confound with strumous and other glandular swellings and mistreat, although they occur in places where there are no glands.

An evidence of this I find in many patients who have sought and obtained help from me, not only after the injurious treatment of the physiological school, but also after unsuccessful Homœopathic treatment.

For the sake of brevity I will only give as much of the correspondence as appertains to the case.

October 16th. "The rheumatic tensive pain on the left side of the neck, the painfulness of the third left rib and of the spinous processes of two of the lumbar vertebræ to pressure, the reddish tubercular eruptions between the scrotum and the thigh of the right side, the sighing respiration, the tearful mood despairing of cure, the œdematous swelling of the feet have all disappeared.

"The following symptoms are relieved: the pressing pain in the shoulders, the painfulness of the hand on grasping and lifting even small objects; the painfulness of the elbow-joint when strongly flexing it, the paralytic weakness of the left leg, in consequence of which it is somewhat easier to rise from a seat and sit down again; the reddish tubercular eruptions of the head and neck, and the sensation as if in the right shoulder a fibre was suddenly torn and jerked loose. Osseous distention of the left parietal bone along the sagittal suture, with less sensitiveness to outward pressure, which symptom I forgot to give in my last letter. The abscess on the right arm near the axilla, which broke once, discharged pus, then healed, has now disappeared by absorption.

"I must add that in the morning and during the forenoon the pains in my leg are relieved, and that the swelling of the knees, especially of the right knee, has disappeared, and that my legs feel best while lying in bed. As I suffered one evening from a violent burning, tearing and itching in the painful eruption at the anus, I resorted to the external use of *Thuja* by which not only was the pain relieved but the condylomata were also reduced at least one third.

"I could not for a moment believe my complaint to be of a sycotic nature, for living twenty-seven years in happy wedlock I have always led a pure life; it would have been a bare impossibility for me to have indulged in sexual intercourse with any other woman.

"One symptom which I have had for many years has become aggravated—a creaking of the ankle when stretching out the foot, so that I am obliged to keep the foot quiet in the joint and have to lie down, whereupon the pain soon leaves. The roaring in my head and ears, which has become habitual, is also much aggravated. To this is added a dullness of the brain which does not, however, interfere with conversation."

To the question whether he should continue the former prescription and might drink beer, I replied in the affirmative.

October 31st. "The tubercular eruption has, for the most part, disappeared; the condylomata (?) at the anus are reduced to the merest trace.

The painfulness of the metacarpal bones on flexing the hand has disappeared. The exostosis on the left parietal bone is much improved, and the pains in the right ankle when stepping have not been noticed for eight days.

"Present condition. Difficulty of hearing and roaring in the head and ears; painfulness of both trochanters and femurs when lying on them. Weakness of the knees as from relaxation of the ligaments; painful cracking of the right ankle when extending it; pain in the right heel when stepping on it; painfulness of the shoulders, of the point of the right elbow and of the right index and ring fingers on pressure; of the left humerus when bending the arm backward, or when raising or extending it. Sensation of stiffness and sleepiness of the hand, especially when resting on the elbow. Pains in the neck when bending the head back. Suppuration of the left axillary gland which is still somewhat hard. Fourteen days ago this was the case in the right axilla. Painful glandular knots in the groins and the anterior surface of the thigh as well as in both sides of the neck. Difficulty of falling asleep; stools insufficient; apparent inactivity of the rectum when at stool, with protrusion of the hæmorrhoids and burning pains; blood when at stool; urine often interrupted, also with a double stream as if from stricture.

"On the whole an improvement in my condition cannot be denied so that I indulge a hope again that I shall be able to resume my practice."

I directed him that if there were any strictures in the urethra they should be dilated, and that otherwise he should continue with *Thuja* and *Nat. sulph.*

November 10th. "Two days after sending my letter the pains in the throat, which had previously disappeared, returned again and light grey ulcers with red edges presented themselves. In my anxiety I took on my own responsibility in place of *Thuja, Lycopod.* 200, several pellets in a tumbler of water, a spoonful morning and evening. *Nat. sulph.* I have continued to take. It is a great remedy. There is nothing worse for me than my own treatment. Since yesterday I have taken morning and evening two drops of *Nitr. acid*, as the ulcers on the throat seem to be spreading again. I expect nothing whatever from *Thuja*. But the symptoms and pains of the leg are considerably better, as well as those of the upper extremities. My mind is active, but without application or endurance, and when reading I am dull and unobservant, yet am in good spirits again.

"Years ago I tried to insert a bougie into the urethra but had to refrain from too great sensitiveness of the passage.

"I shall await your prescription and shall take a dose of *Nitr. ac.* 200, if anything."

I replied: "It would have been better if you had not taken *Nit. ac.* and *Lycop.*; they will do no good. Hold fast to *Thuja* and *Nat. sul.* Whatever may occur, there is no indication whatever for any other course."

November 23rd. "To-day I can report a

great improvement, for the pains in my bones are reduced to a minimum: the knee-joints are stronger so that I can rise much more easily from my seat, and that with the help of one hand only. The pain in the heel is much relieved, and for many days I have experienced such a sense of comfort that while lying in bed where I have otherwise been in the habit of reading, I give myself up entirely to this delightful sense of returning health and do nothing.

"For several days there has been a feeling of some overwork and inclination to sweat, and after I had taken the first dose of *Nat. sul.* yesterday morning I had a pain in the bowels as from diarrhœa; after the second and third dose there appeared besides trembling and fermentation in the bowels. My good appetite was entirely gone at noon. Hence these were effects of *Nat. sul.*, which I have now taken fifty-three days continuously. Thus for the present I have discontinued the remedy. The next evening there was heat in my right ear, chilliness, and when out of bed a shaking chill with increased thirst. Pulse 104. At night slight sweat and good sleep. Pulse now in the morning 116, otherwise I feel well. The sores in the throat have not spread. Since I took *Thuja* again the condylomata have disappeared to a mere trace. My tongue is coated white; the taste is flat; dryness and heat in the mouth; disgust for meat; this morning no colic; eruptions of the forehead and head entirely gone. Since the urethra is no longer as sensitive as it was I have undertaken its dilatation. The urine passes more easily and there is but seldom a double stream. The urinary difficulties are also less. The stricture is situated far back at the entrance of the urethra into the bladder.

"Till further orders I shall suspend the use of Glauber's Salts (*Nat. sul.*), but shall continue with the *Thuja*, which I last took in the 200th (Jenichen's)."

To this I replied: "Since you are now saturated with the Glauber's Salts, you should, as a matter of course, suspend their use for about eight or fourteen days. But I should rather see you continue with *Thuja* 30, for the 200th requires to be taken at longer intervals, otherwise you would have your blood over-saturated with it too soon."

December 24th. "I had already taken *Thuja* 200 at longer intervals but returned to the *Thuja* 30 (four drops) as soon as I received your letter. However, my regular morning stool soon became so hard that I took only two drops. In a few days the stools were easier, but soon after the same difficulties at stool returned again. The stool occurred now with the greatest effort, and was accompanied with burning sore pains lasting all day, so I was obliged to cease the use of *Thuja* entirely, and even at the risk of your finding fault again, I took *Nux vom.* 30 several successive evenings with this result: The stools were passed with more ease, the protruding hæmorrhoids became softer and smaller, and I was no longer annoyed with pain after stool. After ceasing the use of *Thuja* for six days I took it again, but the difficulty at stool returned again at once, so that I resolved to dispense with it for a longer time.

"After having discontinued the *Nat. sul.* for ten days I took it again, three drops in water every hour. After taking it three weeks my appetite diminished again, and last evening also I had a slight chill. I took this to be another indication that I was over-saturated with *Nat. sul.*, and hence will wait for further directions before I take any more medicine.

"In other respects I improve constantly. The pains in my right heel have disappeared entirely, and my legs are so strong again that to-day I was able to rise from my seat without the support of my hands. An enlarged gland in the left groin, which I have noticed for many years, has already diminished very much and become softer, and the kernels on the thigh also appear to grow smaller. In the urethra I can already pass a catheter of large size. The stream of urine is stronger and not divided as before. The eruption on the ears has healed. If I find that I continue to improve, can I take a short walk out of doors? For four months I have not been able to leave the room."

Answer. "There is nothing to be said against the use of intercurrent remedies if they seem necessarily indicated, since you now seem to have lost the hasty anxiety which sometimes leads to things superfluous.

"I now commit to you the further treatment of the case and see no reason why you should not go out in mild weather, if you only guard against too rapid change of temperature.

April 12th. "My disease is so much improved already that I am able to visit patients even several hours distant, and can go up stairs though with some effort. The tubercles are somewhat diminished, the bloody stools as well as the condylomata above the anus have disappeared.

"I have not had any more occasion for intercurrent remedies. *Thuja* and *Nat. sul.* I still use according to your directions."

June 23rd. I received another letter from this colleague asking my advice about one of his patients, with the remark that he was entirely well and could take quite long walks without injury.

[Many years ago, Dr. Pascal of Paris, gave an account of Grauvogl's constitutions in the *Bulletin de l'Homœopathie* and he added to Grauvogl's cases the following which he translated from the Italian *Revista Omiopatica.*—J.H.C.]

DR. GIOVANNI URBANETTI'S CASE.

Hydrogenoid Constitution. Nux, Ipec., Nat. sul.

M.N., 46, tall and well built, having come to Venice with his family in July, 1874, to take the baths, came to consult me and gave me the following account of his case :

"Although my constitution, as you perceive, is neither weak nor delicate, I cannot say I am satisfied with my health. I have never had serious illnesses but I am subject to a crowd of little discomforts which rob me of gaiety, activity and spring, I am very often tormented with coryzas which easily spread to the throat and cause a little difficulty in swallowing, thickening of the voice and bronchial catarrh. I am worried with rheumatic pains though not severe. My digestion is capricious, sometimes good, sometimes bad with bad taste in the mouth. I am *worse in Winter when the weather is cloudy and when it rains. I am always very chilly* and my *feet are constantly rather cold.* I am *better in Summer, and especially when I perspire* I feel relieved; and if by misfortune the sweat is checked I am easily taken with slight shivers and quickly fall back into my usual state of depression. My urine is abundant and the colour varies according as my sufferings are more or less attenuated. I cannot name any likely cause for this state, since my life is very regular, I have never had any suspect maladies, nor has my *morale* had to undergo any violent troubles. The Homœopathic remedies which I take or have prescribed for me, promptly relieve me, it is true, but they do not protect me against frequent and extremely easy relapse. I should like to know from you, sir, if there is any means of establishing my health by any radical treatment whatever?"

To anyone who knows the Constitutions of Grauvogl I imagine it would be impossible to find a more exact picture of the Hydrogenoid Constitution than this. After the directions of the author the indications for the correction of this form of constitution would be:

First, to *restore the spent animal heat ;* then, to *disburden the blood of the excess of hydrogen.* The first result was obtained by exciting the spinal nervous system by *Nux,* and the great sympathetic by *Ipecac.* These two remedies should be given alternately, in a low dilution, frequently through the day and kept up until the bodily heat is restored. The first effect gained, *Nat. sul.* 6, two drops night and morning for a long time to free the organism from the excess of hydrogen, which is the cause of the catarrhs and rheumatism.

After having well studied the symptom picture of this case the choice of these remedies was clearly justified by the law of similars, a guide of which Homœopaths must never lose sight, just as he should never forget the special action of the remedies in high and low dilution, which constitutes a great difference. According to Grauvogl, the low dilutions act more particularly on the organs, tissues and systems affected, whilst the high ones act by preference on the general symptoms.

This is the plan I prescribed for my patient, who promised to follow it out exactly.

In July of the following year he came to see me again and told me the result of the treatment had been very happy. He had passed an exceedingly severe winter in Paris without experiencing any inconvenience.

Chapter VI

EXAMPLES OF THE HYDROGENOID SYCOTIC CONSTITUTION FROM THE PRACTICE OF DR. BOJANUS.

The *North American Journal of Homœopathy* of August and following months, 1888, published a series of cases treated by Dr. Bojanus of Moscow, and published in a German journal. The articles were translated from the German by Dr. T. M. Strong.

Tho first eight of Dr. Bojanus' cases I have somewhat condensed from his narrative. The rest are given in his own words and are written in the first person. The opening of his article runs as follows :

" If in reference to the various constitutions I give preference to the Hydrogenoid, which I shall endeavour to illustrate by examples, I do this chiefly, first, since this constitution for many years past is the predominant one and affords me more material for illustration, and secondly, because it gives practical proof of what Grauvogl says in his posthumous work concerning the subject. May it encourage the study of the works of this eminent and well-deserving enquirer !

" Ever since I began to apply the study of the doctrine of constitutions to practice, and with eminent success—twenty years ago—only one single case of perfect Oxygenoid Constitution has come to my observation.

"The Carbonitrogenoid indeed often appears together with the Hydrogenoid, but seldom alone, and presents in this fashion an extremely difficult, often enigmatically mixed up, therapeutic subject. Almost all of the cases mentioned here belong to the period of time previous to my acquaintance with the posthumous work of Grauvogl; the practical results, of which but a small portion is communicated here, are based chiefly on the study of Grauvogl's *Text-book* and familiar remarks which I have gathered during my acquaintance and conversation with him."

Dr. Bojanus' remarks on the frequent combination and complication of the Hydrogenoid and Carbo-nitrogenoid Constitutions I can fully corroborate, but for all that, the three-fold division can be of great assistance in the selection of remedies. Bojanus endorses what Grauvogl says about the accessory circumstances characterising the constitutions, but the "Constitution" itself is not sufficiently clearly characterised in its exterior manifestations to admit of an exact description of it. "But in reference to the various materials constituting the diet it will be found invariably that aquatic plants and animals, fruits and vegetables largely containing aqueous material—cucumbers, melons, mushrooms, moreover, milk in every form, eggs even cooked soft; as also a moist atmosphere, humidity in dwelling apartments, even accidental and transitory baths, warm or cold, drinks of water or of liquids containing much water; rain, cold, storms, whose approach many persons of this sort feel and foretell in advance, not only may aggravate the disease (in a Nitrogenoid the reverse takes place—at the approach of and during the tempest they feel better), but may also cause a relapse after a disappearance of several months.

"After a complete cure even, the diet restriction should be followed for a further year at least. Among patients of this class some will be able to digest some of the forbidden articles and not others without detriment to their health. Some can take salt-water fish and not fresh-water fish. Some can take eggs and milk but no fish. Most are decidedly averse to flesh meat."

Bojanus gives a very graphic description of the terribly unhygienic condition of Moscow and its two rivers in his day, which mightily fostered the hydrogenoid state in the inhabitants. Filth and ice in winter, dust in summer, floods in spring, and smells all the year round are about the sum of his description. It is not to be wondered at that intermittents are among the endemic diseases he had to treat, and "intermittent fever" and "hydrogenoid constitution" are frequently more or less identical.

I will now give a brief account of Bojanus' cases :

Case I.

Insanity with Intermittent Fever. Veratrum *and* Arsenicum.

O.K., 23, a young lady of an impoverished noble family, whose mother was an energetic lady of strong will, scrofulous in childhood and often subject to neuralgia, dying after her tenth confinement of typhus. The daughter, who was an exact likeness of her mother and very lean and pale, had recently filled a position in Moscow to which she had to make a long journey every day to her office, and lodged in a cold, damp, unwholesome house, where even the bedclothes were hardly ever dry. In childhood she had scrofulous inflammation of the eyes, at thirteen prolonged tinea capitis with large swelling of the neck and its glands. In her fifteenth year the menses appeared for the first time, scanty and always with pains in the abdomen. Three years later leucorrhœa appeared with continual chilliness.

In July, 1875, she left Moscow and went to her father's house twelve miles in the country. At the time Bojanus was called in, August 6th, symptoms of insanity appeared and soon intermittent fever, two paroxysms a day, 10 a.m. to 12 noon, and 8 p.m. to 12 midnight. She was sleepless, continually singing, jumping out of bed and walking up and down the room. There was short interruption of the mania on August 10th ; but the fever continued to return twice a day, and for eight days there was complete sleeplessness, and the singing went on continuously for twenty-four hours on eight occasions, followed by complete aphonia. Pains in the left hypochondrium with enlargement of the spleen were added. *Verat.* 3 was given night and morning and *Arsen.* 3, every three hours during the day. Under these there was steady improvement. By the middle of October the insanity had disappeared, and by November 14th she was well and the remedies were discontinued.

Then followed a relapse brought on by the use of water. During this day, November 14th, she ordered the floor of her room to be scrubbed and as it was not oiled it retained water enough to keep it moist for a long while. Without any apprehension of evil she spent a part of the day and the whole night in that room. At 11 p.m. on the following day she began to complain of headache and pains in the left hypochondrium. There returned also chilliness, weeping, outbursts of temper with terrible excitement and despair about her condition with desire for a speedy death. *Verat.* and *Arsen.* were immediately given in hourly alternation. The next paroxysm appeared at the same hour but was very light, with some sensation of chilliness but without any other inconvenience, and after the 18th all trouble had ceased.

Case II.

Intermittent fever in the form of Congestion of the Brain. Atropine *and* Nat. sulph., *later* Nux *and* Ipec.

Z.B., 6, of cheerful disposition, having had no severe illness, was taken ill 7 a.m. one morning in January, 1871. She awoke screaming, tossing wildly in bed, vacant, glassy stare, pupils dilated, face flushed, pulse slow. Talked absently, imagined strange things, could not be quieted. This lasted an hour and a half, when she fell asleep. Slept till morning, when she awoke and remembered all that had happened. Gentle perspiration set in and she became bright and cheerful. The following day and night there was no complaint, but the second night the same symptoms re-appeared. *Atropine* 6x, and *Nat. Sulph.* 2x, hourly in alternation. Paroxysms recurred but with less intensity. She always remembered what had happened on awaking. After the third night there was no return.

The following year she had scarlet fever in a mild form. All went well till during the desquamation period fever set in. She did not complain of her head or stomach. Thirst increased, sleepless, and when she did sleep muttered and seemed restless. Was constipated and feverish. *Acon.* alone and later *Bellad.* were without effect. Then careful observations showed that there were intermissions and Bojanus concluded that it was the old intermittent that he had to deal with. *Arsen.* every three hours was given, water was forbidden as drink unless mixed with wine. From this time the fever diminished and in ten days she was well, but *Arsen.* was continued at increased intervals until the twenty-first day.

After this Z.B. had good health for several months when it was noticed that she had a short but continual cough while sleeping. It lasted several nights but ceased between 4 and 5 a.m. *Cham.*, *Nux*, *Hyos.* and several other remedies were given without effect before

Bojanus was called in. He then recognised that it was merely another form of the original complaint. There was rough bronchial breathing in the left side and posteriorly. *Nux.* and *Ipecac.* were given every three hours alternately with the anti-hydrogenous diet and in a week she was free from cough. At fourteen she had measles lightly, she menstruated for the first time and since then was in perfect health. She was twenty-two when Bojanus wrote.

Case III.

Intermittent in the form of Meningitis. Atropine 6x *and* Nat. sulph.

Adele W., 10, tall, slender, pale, hollow-chested, delicate, was out walking one clear day in March, 1881, and on returning home suddenly complained of being sick. Her symptoms were : raging headache, severe chill followed by intense heat, intolerance of light, very nervous, nausea, vomiting first food then bile. The following night very restless, dozed a little but on awaking always had headache, at times slightly delirious.

Next morning she was very feverish, high temperature, raging headache, loud singing noise in ears, convulsive twitching of muscles of face, especially about mouth and cheeks, very sensitive to touch and irritated by the least noise.

Bellad. 3x was given every hour. Next day no change. The day after, March 4th, much better. *Bellad.* was continued and hydrogenous diet ordered. On March 7th she was taken with severe chills which lasted fully three days. It was now clear that it was a question of an intermittent. *Atrop. sul.* 6x and *Nat. sul.* 2x, of each three drops was given on wafers, the body to be rubbed with spirits, and water only to be drunk mixed with wine. On March 14th she had another paroxysm in a light form and on the 21st another still lighter. From that time she began to recover her health and appetite and grew stout.

In March, 1882, one night she went to bed well and woke up in a few hours screaming with pain in right ear, cheeks flushed, more on right side. *Atrop.* 6x. Next two days she was free from pain but on the fourth day she had another attack but less severe. *Atrop.* 6x, and *Nat. sul.* 2x every hour. There were four more attacks, all quartan and each time shorter and lighter. She was seen last in the winter of 1884 when she was well and had been so since the last attack.

Case IV.

Intermittent Fever in the form of Lepto-meningitis.
Nux *and* Belladonna, Nat. sul. *and* Nux.
(I give this case in Bojanus' own words. J.H.C.)

In January, 1870, a distinguished gentleman called on me and invited me to visit his sick child, who, he said, had been under the care of three physicians, one of them being Professor F., of Moscow University, whose speciality was children's diseases.

I learned from the father that his daughter was three years old, had been ill six weeks, and the doctors had told him his daughter was suffering from inflammatory hydrocephalus. I remember having then made the remark that there must be an error somewhere, for from my experience, and from what I had read, I had never heard of so protracted a case of lepto-meningitis. When I arrived at midnight I found the child lying on her right side, her face turned to the wall and her right hand resting under her cheek; her legs were crossed; she was asleep but eyes partly open; she was very thin and pale; her skin not warm, but normal; she was breathing easily; pulse, 80-90, not hard; would cry at the least touch. I found between the two shoulder-blades a blister the size of the hand due to a vesicant. This I immediately opened and applied a cerate dressing.

While I was doing this she cried, but showed no other abnormal signs. She was very much constipated. With the best of good will I could not find out how those physicians made such a diagnosis. The intelligent nurse said it was but natural I should think so as I had not seen her when she had her spells, but if I would take the trouble to call the next morning about eight o'clock I should probably agree with them. On further questioning the nurse she told me that the child's mother, who was still a young woman and nursing her youngest child, through sorrow and trouble had nearly lost her mind.

At first the child's sickness attacked her in spells, but each day she became worse ; to-day she had a quiet one, but to-morrow, at the same time, would become worse ; her sickness would begin with cold hands and feet and headache, vomiting of bilious matter, squinting and rolling her eyes, with convulsive motions of the face and occasionally of the extremities. This would last for three hours, then she would become more quiet, and by the afternoon and during the next day would be in her usual health.

I now examined the liver and spleen, and found the left lobe of the liver enlarged to the extent of one and a half finger-breadths, and the spleen to an equal if not greater extent ; chalk-white stool (similar to what might occur from an exclusive milk diet) without any icteric taint. Urine dark and without sediment ; appetite poor and only on the well days ; lived almost exclusively on milk which she also took to satisfy her thirst.

I informed the parents that under the circumstances I might not be able to group properly all the conditions, but no time should be lost on this account, since everything pointed to one conclusion, that we were not dealing with an acute hydrocephalus. On the next morning at 7 o'clock I went to see the child in order to see the symptoms reported by the parents. A few minutes before eight o'clock the hands and feet became cold, followed by pale face, headache and weeping, the latter occasionally interrupted by a shrill cry. Twice there was a slight vomiting of bilious matter. After this condition had lasted over one hour the cheeks began to redden, the temperature increased to 39.3C, pulse 100 to 120, occasionally intermittent, generally full, eyes distorted, twitching in the face with drawing of the mouth as if in laughter, pupils contracted, respiration quickened, intelligence lessened, slight convulsive movement of the left side. Half an hour later the child began to bore the head into the pillow, while there was at the same time a convergent squint. There was no more vomiting, but at intervals a shrill cry. The paroxysm lasted until 11.30 a.m., when amelioration began, so that by 1 p.m. the condition was nearly normal. *Nux* 3x and *Bellad.* 3x, two drops every two hours in alternation were given; milk and water were forbidden and only wine and water with a little sugar were allowed as drink. The body to be rubbed with 90° spirits.

To compel obedience to these rules was very difficult, since there was but one opinion under the circumstances, namely, that the case was a most desperate if not hopeless one. After many unsuccessful remonstrances I finally said that since the child had been given up by the physicians we could only try, and that I could not permit any other treatment than the one ordered and if not permitted to carry it out unrestricted I would cease attendance.

This had the desired effect, the nurse obeyed my orders accurately. I gave the child an injection of warm water to relieve the constipation.

I called about eight o'clock the next morning,

thinking she would have another spell, which attacked her at nine o'clock, but in the same way, namely, with cold hands and feet, and she begged to have more covering over her (which she had not asked for before).

She also had a severe headache, but did not scream. Soon after she became feverish, with a temperature of 38.5C, pulse 80 to 85. She was not delirious and had no convulsive movements of face or extremities. She then fell asleep until 10 o'clock, and perspired freely which she had not done before. She awakened about one o'clock, was very weak and indifferent. Soon followed a pale, grass-green stool. The three following paroxysms, still of the tertian type, did not differ in intensity or duration, except that the perspiration was decidedly less. Apparently there was a change in the condition. Since improvement went on slowly, and the lessened perspiration seemed to threaten a relapse, in place of the *Belladonna* I gave *Natrum sulphuricum* 2x in alternation with the *Nux* 3x, every two hours. After this she had two paroxysms accompanied by profuse prespiration. The second, however, was light, and after this the child began to recover; appetite and sleep improved and by continuing the use of the remedies, but not so often, until the twenty-eighth day after having the last paroxysm, and with a strict diet, in three weeks she was able to leave her bed and walk about.

In 1876 I saw her for the last time. She was then in good health and I have not heard from her since.

An interesting part of this case is that when the child was able to go about the father met Prof. F. in the street, when the Professor inquired after the child. On being told that she was well, he threw up his hands above his head and exclaimed, "That is impossible!" "Come and see her and satisfy yourself," replied the father. But he did not come.

Case V.

Neuralgia, Chill, Night-cough. Nux. *and* Arsenicum, Nux. *and* Ipecac.

Frau E. von E., a slender delicate woman of good constitution, who celebrated her eightieth birthday during her illness, complained in December, 1863, of pain in the left side of the face, especially in the zygoma, the pain being of a tearing, drawing nature. The corner of the mouth was slightly drawn to the left, and there was twitching of the lower eyelid. There were marked remissions and occasional intermissions which were very irregular. There was no periodicity noticed. The pain was markedly < at night. In other respects the patient was perfectly well and actively busy with her usual duties. *Spigelia* 12, three drops every two hours, was prescribed, and the pain gradually disappeared, only the twitching of the lower eyelid remaining. *Causticum* was now given night and morning, and a few days later the twitching was gone.

But this was succeeded by a severe chill lasting the entire day and followed in the evening by high fever which continued the whole night. This produced complete loss of appetite, but did not affect the general health and she continued at work as before. *Causticum* was continued, but as there was no change at the end of a week, a wine diet and rubbing the body with brandy were ordered and *Nux.* 3x and *Arsen.* 3x were given every two hours alternately.

At the end of a week the feverish condition had lessened, but a night cough, entirely relieved by day, now came on. Otherwise her condition remained the same except that her appetite was better. The loss of sleep weakened her and although she got some sleep in the day it did not make up for that lost in the night. *Nux* 3x and *Ipec.* 3x were now given every two hours alternately. In a few days the cough disappeared, the sleep returned and the patient seemed well. Several weeks later when Bojanus again called she told him that after the cough left she had been weak and then noticed a swelling in the back of the feet which had increased slowly till it reached the knees. She complained only of difficulty in walking and itching of the swollen extremities and was otherwise well. There was a trace of albumen in the urine but no casts, and liver and spleen were normal. Bojanus ordered a half lemon to be taken night and morning with plenty of sugar but no water. At the end of a week the œdema was gone and the patient was not again ill till she died of old age at 88.

Case VI.

Intermittent Fever under the form of Prosopalgia.
Nux *and* Ipec., *later* Aranea.

D.B., wife of a Russian clergyman, 36, small of stature, emaciated and badly nourished, mother of several children, consulted Bojanus on March 6th, 1878, complaining of pain in the left side of the face, which was of long duration and came on every day at 2 p.m. It followed the three branches of the trigeminus, and she also complained of a persistent chilliness not relieved by the heat of the sun or a warm room. This had lasted two years, the pain in the face having first appeared in March, 1877, and had proved intractable to all kinds of household remedies and was only removed by *Quinine* given under medical advice. But the general health was not improved, and in the beginning of autumn the pain returned and though again relieved by *Quinine* the relief was slower in coming than at first. She now gave this history :

With the onset of chilliness, with cold hands and feet, there appears a burning pain deep in behind the joint of the lower jaw. The pain radiates into the eye causing weeping, into the eyelids, the left side of the nose, the cheek and all the teeth, upper and lower and even to the chin and lips. To this pain there is added a particularly painful, intermittent tearing sensation from within outwards. The only relief was by the application of very hot dry cloths. After the attack had lasted about two hours the pains began to slowly lessen, the entire attack lasting from three to three and a half hours, after which she felt very weak and faint. Fever and sweating were absent during the attack. She complained of want of appetite, the tongue was coated white with insipid taste, and there was aversion to meat; long continued sensations of coldness or chilliness over the whole body and constant coldness of the hands and feet. The liver and spleen were normal, menses regular and scanty but without pain, no constipation or thirst. *Nux* 3x and *Ipec.* 3x were given every hour in alternation during the pains. The usual diet and wine were ordered and no water except mixed with wine. On March 17th she reported that after three days the pains began to disappear gradually and for three days there had not been any, but the chilliness and cold hands and feet remained. On April 26th, the pain had not returned and the chilliness and cold hands were better, as also the general health.

The medicines were continued at longer intervals with strict instructions that the diet should be continued for at least one year. On March 28th, 1879, the patient reported that the pains had returned one week before. Since April 1878, she had taken the medicines as ordered, for two weeks four times daily, in alternation, for two weeks twice and for a further two weeks once a day. But she had not been strict with the diet, especially in the latter part of the time. Nevertheless, she had been in good health until the beginning of the great fast (Lent). (According to the laws of the Russian Church the seven weeks of the fast are very strictly kept. Nothing but vegetable food is allowed; only on two days of this long fast can fish be eaten, namely, at the feast of the Annunciation and Palm Sunday. The diet consists of cabbages, turnips, potatoes, mushrooms and farinacious foods, everything being prepared with oil; animal food is strictly excluded.) Believing that she was quite well she began to fast and at first suffered no inconvenience, but on March 25th she could not resist the desire for fish and on the 26th the neuralgia returned, together with the coldness of the hands and feet. It also transpired that since the winter she had been living in a very damp house. *Aranea* 3x and *Spigelia* 3x were given in hourly alternation.

On April 12th the pains had been entirely absent for three days and the patient felt decidedly better. The remedies were continued and it was directed that for twenty-eight days after the last attack the diet should be strictly observed and a drier dwelling found. Seen by Bojanus when attending her children during 1882 to 1884 there had been no return of the trouble.

Case VII.

Intermittent Fever under the form of Pneumonia. Ipecac. *and* Nux.

B.T., 4, a well-nourished, strong, active boy, was taken ill on January 10th, 1875. The previous day he had given a few coughs, which had passed unnoticed, but about 2 a.m. he was suddenly seized with a severe shaking chill, followed in an hour with high fever and reddened cheeks. He was restless, continually tossing about, coughed frequently and cried continually from pain in the chest, but was unable to locate the seat. After this had lasted two and a half hours sweating began and the cough lessened, crying ceased and the boy soon fell asleep. The sweating continued, though not copious, till 9 a.m., when he awoke without any distress and after eating his breakfast, went to his accustomed playing. So passed twenty-four hours and again a slight cough occurred, almost unnoticed by the parents and not attended to. Soon after midnight of the 12th occurred the same scene, and in the morning of the 13th Bojanus saw the child. As soon as he entered the dwelling he noticed that it was damp, which the parents admitted and said that they were determined to leave it in the spring. The boy was then up and busy with his playthings, without any special appearance of sickness.

Examination showed that there was no fever. The tongue was slightly coated and there had been no stool since the day before. Percussion gave negative results. There were fine bubbling râles under the left scapula; when quiet there was no cough, but it at once appeared when moving about. Bojanus diagnosed bronchitis or catarrhal pneumonia with a malarial complication and warned the parents that they might expect another paroxysm. *Ipec.* 3x, in two-drop doses, was given every hour.

The next paroxysm came on at 10 p.m., and was ushered in with a severe chill, which lasted one hour, and great thirst; the cough quickly followed and was accompanied with headache and general pain, together with restless tossing about the bed. A few minutes after eleven the fever began with reddened cheeks, increased heart-action and a temperature of 39.3 to 39.9C. There was quicker respiration, violent action of the nostrils, drawing in of the lower ribs, aggravation of the cough, increased restlessness, crying and tossing around, all continuing until half-past twelve. The thirst was not so great during the fever. The child became easier as the sweating stage began, which was this time more copious and of shorter duration than in the previous attacks, the whole paroxysm being lighter, as the mother said, than the former ones.

Nux. 3x and *Ipec.* 3x were given in hourly alternations during the interval, together with wine diet and rubbing morning and evening with brandy. The three following paroxysms were each lighter in character and after the last the child began to improve rapidly. During the Spring and early Summer he was well and before the hot weather was removed to a drier dwelling and then into the country, so that he suffered neither a relapse nor a new attack. Seen in 1884, then fourteen years old, he was in rugged health and had had no other sickness.

Case VIII.

Intermittent Fever under the form of Pleurisy.

Nux. *and* Ipec.; Ipec. *and* Aranea.

M.D., 46, mother of a grown-up daughter, had suffered for many years on each recurring spring with the following conditions :

Early in March, without any visible cause, she would be attacked with a severe sticking pain in the left side of the chest which interfered with the respiration and with this there was a chilly feeling lasting an hour, followed by fever lasting three hours, during which the pains were aggravated, the breathing more difficult, and accompanied with a cough, generally without expectoration, but sometimes there was a frothy, slimy sputum. There was also intense thirst, dryness of the mouth, headache and internal chilliness but with hot skin with desire to be covered during this period and sometimes longer, sometimes shorter but never of over three hours duration. This was followed by profuse sweating lasting generally from two to two and a half hours, during which the pains lessened, the breathing became freer and the cough looser. On the following day the patient was able to be up for a few hours, but this only lasted two days when the attack recurred. This state of things lasted till May, when every symptom disappeared and she gradually recovered her health.

The usual treatment gave no relief. The only benefit she got was from *Quinine*, but latterly she had been compelled to take such large doses that they caused a feeling of apprehension and giddiness. Bojanus found the general condition on the whole discouraging: appetite poor, cannot take milk which causes diarrhœa, nor fish, which causes pain in the stomach and nausea; she does not care for uncooked fruit and has an aversion to meat, so that, as she expressed it, eating is a matter of indifference. She was emaciated, often compelled to resort to wine, spoke slowly and in measured tones, always felt weak and exhausted. The tongue was slightly coated, no constipation, sleep generally light, disinclination to motion and work which she ascribed to her weakness.

In March, 1876, an examination, Bojanus writes, showed the following: "Liver normal, spleen slightly sensitive to pressure. Percussion gave negative results, while auscultation showed, with normal respiration, at the sixth intercostal space on the left and backwards a distinctly audible friction sound, so distinct, indeed, that I was not certain of its cause. This much was certain, that we had to deal with a quartan type of intermittent fever. *Nux* 3x and *Ipec.* 3x, three drops of each were given in hourly alternation together with a wine diet and rubbing of the whole body with alcohol three times daily. At the next attack all the symptoms returned and I heard during the fever paroxysm the friction sound under the before-mentioned painful spot. For this I ordered a compress to be applied during the fever, removing it when the sweating stage came on. After four successive lessening attacks the fifth failed to appear and the patient began to improve. The appetite increased, also the general strength and she became more active and in better spirits. Auscultation showed steady vesicular respiration and complete absence of the friction sound. A few weeks later the patient went to the country with instructions to continue the medicine and closely follow the diet.

"During the following winter she enjoyed good health but in the early part of April I was again called to see her, and learnt that the attacks had returned, but in a tertian form, although she could not remember any error of diet and the attacks were somewhat different; she has now constant chilliness, the fever and pain in the side were less and the paroxysms did not last as long. I again examined during the paroxysm, percussion gave no results and I heard on auscultation, distinct normal respiration and a very slight friction sound. She now received *Ipec.* 3x and *Aranea* 3x in hourly doses, together with the same diet and rubbing with spirit. The second attack was so slight that she had no desire to remain in bed, and there was no other. In 1880 I saw the patient for the last time, and she had had no sickness up to that time.

[The remaining cases are given in Bojanus' own words.]

CASE IX.

Intermittent in the form of Pleurisy. Nux *and* Ipec.

This case, very similar to the last, says Bojanus, came to me in 1872.

The five-year-old son of General R. had been treated for two weeks by an old-school physician but without benefit. When I saw the child for the first time, a plaster, leaving a blister, had been removed from the affected side so that percussion and auscultation were not to be thought of in this capricious, spoiled and feared-inspired boy, who at the approach of every stranger uttered a terrified cry. I learned from the mother that two weeks before, without any apparent cause, he was attacked by a chill, not long in duration, followed by fever. With the chill he began to cough and with each coughing spell distorted the face and cried. He also complained of pain in the left side, more towards the back. The physician was called and said that the trouble was pleurisy, which was evident enough, and ordered a mixture which was given at once. Soon after this, sweating began and he rested easier, and towards evening of the same day the disease had apparently disappeared, which was naturally ascribed to the mixture. On the next day the boy seemed relatively well and was running round the room since it was impossible to keep him in bed. On the following day the same scene was repeated and so continued until the boy refused to take the medicine and it was not possible to use force. The mixture contained *Quinine*. Up to the time of consulting me the attacks had been of the tertian type. I could not examine nor question the boy, but from his well-nourished and vigorous appearance, and from my own experience, the scrofulous basis was plainly manifest. I gave *Nux* 3x and *Ipec.* 3x in hourly doses, and ordered a wine diet, to which the mother at first objected. During the following week there were three paroxysms of which the third and last was very light, and the boy was soon well. He now permitted a careful examination, but it was without result. For three or four years after this I have seen the boy and during that time there has been no relapse.

Case X.

Long-continued Intermittent Fever, simulating Tuberculosis. Phos., Kali. nit., Nux *and* Arsen.

A young man, 20, of whose family I had been physician for many years, had suffered greatly from intermittent fever the last two years while residing in Dorpat, where he was attending the gymnasium and, as his parents would not employ old school treatment, he was prescribed for by letter, and each time relieved, but from want of perseverance with the diet, and on account of the climatie influence, he was constantly subject to relapses.

In February, 1882, this tall, but reasonably strong young man, of good constitution, again fell sick. When a child he had had scarlatina of rather severe form with albuminuria. Later he had measles but no other diseases, except the above-mentioned intermittent fever whieh frequently relapsed notwithstanding the use of *Nux*, *Arsen.*, *Chinin. arsenicosum* and *Natrum mur.* As he was preparing for his graduation examination he could not return home but was compelled to remain at Dorpat until the end of May. His elder brother was at the same time a student of medieine in Dorpat and could do nothing but eall upon Professor V——, who proeeeded to treat him, *secundum artem*, with large doses of *Quinine* and stopped the paroxysm, but as it persisted in returning, larger doses of the drug were used. So matters went on until he had passed the examination and was about to attempt the matrieulant's examination for the university.

At this time he was seized with a general feeling of exhaustion and an irritating dry eough whieh alarmed his brother, and Professor V—— was again ealled. He made a eareful examination and found dulness with abnormal respiration at the left apex and ordered the patient to seek a warm southern elimate.

Daily towards evening there was fever with copious night-sweats, and in the faee of Professor V——'s opinion already expressed, the brother asked him what he feared. "Dear friend," said the Professor, "here is a serious matter; do you not see that tubereulosis and heetie are in union? I have seen a mass of sueh patients; I am not mistaken."

The young man was startled and eould not believe the words, although they were those of a master, and so ealled in Dr. S——, who, after seeing the patient, gave, if not in the same words, at least the same sentiment, and thus the eorreetness of the diagnosis was established.

The brother now wrote home deseribing *in extenso* the eondition of the patient, as also the result of the physieal examination, whereby it beeame apparent that the fever reeurred every evening with slight ehill, general heat, and a copious sweating, thus simulating hectic fever. I wrote to Dorpat inquiring if the professors thought the condition of the lungs to be a result or cause of the fever, since, if they determined that this was the cause of the fever, then the changes in the lungs must have preceded and not followed the fever, and this the more since it was known to me that these same gentlemen had examined this patient at other times and pronounced the lungs to be in good condition. I was also anxious to have this question answered since they had decided not only in this but in other similar cases, that a rational therapeutic treatment was not possible.

The answer returned was that the fever was a hectic fever and was dependent on a commencing disease in the lung. I saw that my question had not been understood and urged the patient to come to Moscow, which he did. On his arrival I examined him most carefully but could discover no dulness although the abnormal breathing was noticeable. I also learned that for the past three years, in each succeeding Spring, he had suffered from intermittent fever, and during the present season the same, and as it did not seem to yield to the medicines which I had sent, large doses of *Quinine* had been taken up to ten-grain doses. Still the fever returned until finally the attack came on each evening with chill, heat, headache, weakness, despondency, ill-humour, restlessness and dry cough. These conditions were also present, in a lessened degree, during the apyrexia. The young man had grown thin, there was loss of appetite, the sleep was disturbed on account of the fever and night sweats, and was only an unrefreshing slumber, while the normal condition was very much disturbed. I ordered *Phos.* 3x and *Kali nit.* 3x hourly in alternation with the wine diet and rubbing the body with spirits. At the end of three weeks, under the continuous use of these two remedies, the fever and abnormal breathing had entirely disappeared, while the appetite had improved and the patient was cheerful and bright.

In order to quiet the family, and also on hygienic considerations, I advised the young man to seek another climate, and, in order to lose no time, to begin his studies in South Germany, which was done. In the meantime, his brother, who had attained his degree, travelled through Austria in October of the same year and was a witness of his good health and activity in his studies.

In the Spring of 1883 the former wrote me that his brother had had a threatening of a return of the fever but that *Nux* and *Arsen.* promptly relieved it. After spending a year in Austria my patient returned to Dorpat to complete his studies in natural science and philosophy and then travelled. So far as I know, he has not been sick since the occasion noted above.

Case XI.

Sycosis. Nux *and* Ipec.; Thuja, Nat. sul.

Mr. K——, worker in a glove factory, 28, tall and strong, of pale countenance and spare build complained that for one year, especially in the autumn and winter months, he had suffered from a cough, which was accompanied by a constant, generally copious, thick, yellowish or greyish expectoration, which in the last attack was also mingled with blood and this led him to seek advice. According to his report the cough had not come on any single occasion from catching cold. He was not able to give any particulars of his condition except that for a year, or about the time that the cough began, he had gonorrhœa, which had been treated according to the old-school method and had only been cured about a month.

On examination of the genitals I found over twenty narrow-pedicle condylomata about the glans and especially around the corona. Percussion showed marked dulness in the upper part of the left lung extending down into the third intercostal space, while auscultation demonstrated harsh bronchial breathing, which, in every case, points to extensive infiltration. A distant weak vesicular murmur could also be heard in the same side. The third and seventh dorsal vertebræ were sensitive to pressure. The cough, which was < in the morning, was not debilitating. It was caused by a persistent tickling in the throat, which at night interfered with sleep, at which time the cough was drier. His strength was lessened and also his appetite. Cold water, cucumber and water-melon caused a watery, painless diarrhœa, so that only boiled water could be taken and this in the smallest quantity. The stool was sluggish.

There was no fever but lately constant chilliness not > in a warm room.

On November 10th, 1868, he received *Nux* 3x and *Ipec.* 3x, three drops in hourly alternation, and anti-hydrogenoid diet. On December 1st he reported that he was feeling better and that within a week the cough had nearly disappeared. The medicines were continued at intervals of two hours. On December 10th the cough had not returned, the chilliness was better and some of the warts had fallen off the glans; there was an insignificant thin discharge from the urethra; he felt stronger on the whole, his appetite was better and the stool regular. Physical examination of the thorax showed a clearer percussion sound over the affected area, and a somewhat rough, prolonged, but not bronchial breathing; the tenderness over the spine was better. *Thuja* 30 and *Nat. sul.* 2x were now ordered morning and evening.

On January 12th only two of the condylomata remained, the discharge from the urethra had ceased, as also the chilliness, while the appetite, stool and general health were very satisfactory. The remedies were repeated and on February 2nd all the condylomata had gone. The chest showed everywhere normal percussion sound and strong vesicular murmur. The tenderness over the spine was gone, the colour of the skin was good and the patient's former strength, through good appetite and regular digestion, had again returned. No further medicine was given but he was directed to report later. This he did on March 20th and I satisfied myself by a thorough examination of his restoration to health.

CASE XII.

Intermittent Fever and Perihepatitis. Nux 3x *and* Arsen. 3x.

A wealthy lady, 30, mother of two children, who had as a young girl taken for anæmia or chlorosis large quantities of *Iron* in the form of Vallet's pills, and had lost nearly all her teeth in consequence, was taken ill in February, 1868, with a severe chill, accompanied with severe pains in the right hypochondrium and pressure in the stomach which was greatly aggravated by free respiration. This was followed by fever, not intense, lasting several hours and followed by sweating. By this time it was evening, and after spending a bad night with frequently interrupted sleep, she was alarmed to see her skin as well as her eyes had a strong icteric colouration.

From this time these attacks began to manifest themselves in regular tertian type, during which the icterus persisted in its intensity, but the pains in the hypochondrium lessened during the apyrexia; no other symptoms manifested themselves.

The patient was treated up to the beginning of May with old-school measures—soda water, soda baths and many other remedies unknown to me—also with homœopathic remedies, whilst all possible diagnoses were given even to the presence of micrococci, but all without relief.

She then went to Carlsbad. There she drank of the Markt and Muhlbrunnen, and bathed in Sprudelwasser, but the only relief obtained was that the paroxysm ehanged from a tertian to an eight-day attaek. During this long interval the ieterus almost disappeared, although the urine still eontained a large quantity of bile pigment and the fœees retained a white, bile-defieient eolour. After the patient had remained six weeks at Carlsbad without any benefit she beeame impatient and losing hope of any result returned to her home.

I was eonsulted the end of July and found the following eonditions : Very weak and emaeiated, marked ieterie eolour of the skin, with intensely yellow seleræ. The left lobe of the liver was at least three inehes below the borders of the ribs, extending to the serobieulus eordis ; it eould also be traeed baekwards to the middle of the last rib and was very sensitive. The gall-bladder eould be felt as a round elastie body. The spleen seemed to be normal. Over the whole body were seratehed and bleeding spots due to the itehing from the ieterus. The appetite was poor, the tongue eoated, a bitter taste in the mouth, the urine was filled with gall pigment, the fæees ehalk-white, and the menses had not appeared sinee February last. The paroxysm eame on regularly every eight days at the same hour, but on the seventh day the patient felt an oppressed feeling about the heart, aeeompanied with diffieult breathing and an indeseribable diseomfort, due to the approaehing paroxysm. The latter eame on in the morning lasting till evening and began with a light chill, followed immediately with a severe pain of a pressing sticking character in the region of the liver, extending also to the cardiac region causing there an unendurable distress with difficult breathing. The fever was rather severe in character, lasting about one hour, with little thirst but with intense aggravation of the pains about the liver. During this time the liver was so sensitive that the slightest touch could not be endured; the swelling of the liver and distension of the gall bladder were also increased, whilst the sufferings could not be borne without hot applications which afforded manifest relief. This continued until towards evening, when the pains began to abate at the outset of a slight perspiration, so that by ten o'clock the patient was again in a comfortable condition and was only troubled by the increased icterus and persistent itching of the skin. During the seven days' apyrexia the swelling of the liver and gall-bladder and the jaundice of the skin disappeared and the patient was able to move about and take short walks in the garden. No headache or other disturbances were present.

She received *Nux* 3x and *Arsen.* 3x, three drops of each in hourly doses, was ordered wine diet and to have the body rubbed night and morning with alcohol. The next paroxysm, also after an interval of a week, showed itself only by a feeling of weakness and discomfort, and the pains, swelling of the liver, chills and fever were wanting so that the patient was not compelled to lie down nor to apply the hot compresses. On the following day there was a sudden urging to stool, the movement consisting of a partly formed white partly coloured pappy fæcal mass mixed with a partially thick, grass-green, watery fluid of fetid odour. From this time the decrease of the swollen liver was daily evident. The gall-bladder could not be felt on the day following the stool. The icterus slowly disappeared and with it the itching of the skin, while the appetite at the end of two weeks was voracious, and as the restoration of the whole organism went on the patient began to gain flesh, to recover her strength. By the end of August, up to which time the medicines had been continued, but at longer intervals, one would hardly know her. The medicines were given once a day in alternation to the end of September, when they were discontinued. There has been no relapse up to the time of writing.

Case XIII.

Sycosis. Thuja *and* Nat. sul.

Herr von Z——, a feeble young man, 29, of delicate constitution, an officer of artillery, had, in October, 1862, all the symptoms of gonorrhœa, having been exposed to infection, and in addition an ulcer on the glans, which the attending physician at once announced to be syphilitic.

A thorough use of *Mercury* (the preparation unknown to the patient) both internally and externally, healed the ulcer and reduced the acute gonorrhœa to a chronic, painless, insignificant discharge. He was an invalid nearly a month and was discharged near the end of November. During this treatment the health of the patient was much impaired ; he was pale and anæmic, with little appetite, and could not recuperate. In December there was a pustulous eruption on the head, to which he gave no heed. Soon after this he noticed a moist, sometimes painful swelling in the anus, and finally also white spots in the mouth and throat. For all these he treated himself, but without result. He then consulted a physician, who took all these symptoms for secondary syphilis, and in consideration of his anæmic condition gave him *Iodides* ; but as these gave no result, the *Protoiodide of Mercury* was prescribed, with the sole result of producing a profuse salivation. So the *Iodides* were again resorted to. So went the treatment around without any visible improvement until April, 1863. This led him to leave Kasan, where he had lived, and come to Moscow. Here a so-called specialist in secret diseases assured him of an ointment which was a sure cure and would remove all the complaints after *a very small quantity* of the remedy had been used. He made *only* forty applications and some of these to several insignificant mucous plaques on the lips, which nevertheless the specialist affirmed were the after-effects of the ointment already applied. In consideration of his weak condition and the anæmia, as also from wise and secret reasons, the apparently cured one was sent into a warmer climate. On the journey to Italy he was seized in Turin with an angina, and consulting a physician, received large doses of *Sulphate of Soda*, and later *Kali chloricum* internally and *Iodine* externally. He was treated a long time without the slightest improvement in his condition. *Tartar emetic* was then given, but in what doses the patient does not know. A few days after taking this remedy the angina disappeared, as also the mucous plaques with which it was complicated. After this, the now apparently convalescent man spent some time in Italy waiting in vain for the favourable action of the warm climate upon his strength, and then journeyed into Switzerland, where he had another attack of angina. He was treated at a water-cure, with the result of bringing back the mucous patches without relieving the angina. This complete overpowering of the favourable action of *Tartar emetic*, as shown in the cure at Turin, an account of which having been given by the patient, surprised the doctor of the water-cure and made him prove untrue to his principles, so that he prescribed *Tartar emetic* with the same result as before. The again convalescing patient spent the winter of 1863 and the summer of 1864, vainly waiting for returning strength and the disappearance of the anæmia, part of the time being spent in Switzerland and part in Southern France, until September, 1864, when he arrived in Paris. He then suffered from a headache, which he thus described: The pain came in different parts of the head, moved from one side to the other, and was for the most part of a drawing and boring character and seemed to lie deep in the brain.

As the termination of his furlough was drawing near he was prevented, perhaps fortunately, from calling upon a Parisian corypheus and so travelled with his headache.

In the beginning of October, 1864, he came to Moscow and put himself again under the care of the specialist who had formerly treated him. Here he remained until December, being treated with Russian baths and *Iodide*, but without any improvement, but on the contrary with a progressive increase of his distress. On the 9th of December I was called to attend him, and found the following conditions :

Pale, anæmic, wasted almost to a skeleton, he lay in bed being only free from headache during the morning hours. When the headache is on he can neither move, think or collect his thoughts. He answered in a very low tone, loud speaking resounding in the head, so that he presented an appearance of imbecility. He described the headache as deep in the brain, but not located on any one spot, the pain being boring, gnawing, tearing, and so severe as to cause him to rave and wish himself dead. The headache generally begins between 5 and 7 p.m., reaching its height at 12 midnight, and then declining with morning, so that between 7 and 8 a.m. he has the greatest relief. The appetite was poor, the stool torpid, urine normal, the old gonorrhœa still existed in a mild form, with slight discharge and no pain. He slept very little either in the night or during the morning remission. The head pains were greatly < by noise and light. If he was spoken to he answered in a monosyllabic, depressed, weeping manner, hesitating long on his answer, and not always comprehending the question, and when alone he lay as if in a stupor. He was < in damp weather. The only thing which gave him comfort was a temperature of 38 to 40 R. (118-120 F.). This he sought daily in the special room of the Russian baths, nor could he admit any moisture into this room, and the heat gave no relief to the headache.

It should be noted that the above facts were not obtained at my first visit, but later on when he was able to put them in order, since on my first visit his mind could bear only the slightest strain. I gave him *Thuja* 200 in four ounces of water, a teaspoonful morning and evening; whilst during the day he received *Nat. sulph.* 2x, two drops three or four times a day.

The result was so surprising that at the end of one week the headache had improved to such a degree that he was already more active and could now spend the day in comparative comfort. The sleep also returned except just before and after midnight, when he had headache; but it was easily endured, and this disappeared at the end of the second week, the same remedies being continued. After this the appetite returned, and by the 30th December his strength had wonderfully increased. By this time the urethral discharge, which has lasted from the beginning of the illness, was completely removed.

The patient remained in Moscow until January, 1865, continuing the use of the remedies, without any return of the symptoms, and once more he appeared in social life, attending parties, balls and the theatre. At the latter date he went to Kiew, and soon after this he was married. Two years later I heard that he was a father, and had never had a return of his former conditions.

Case XV.

Sycosis.—Arsen. *and* Nux; Thuja *and* Nat. sul.

N.N., 38, an old-school physician in Taroslaw, presented, on February 25th, 1869, the following conditions: A small man, spare, wan, of weak constitution, had noticed for nearly a year a swelling near the right sacral bone which measured near its base 11 c.m. broad and 14 c.m. long, and 1 c.m. high. It was surrounded by a hard, immovable, not everywhere equally thick margin, with distinct fluctuation, so that by touch its form could be determined and the presence of fluid ascertained. The margin had the consistency of a hardened gland and simulated the latter in not having the same thickness everywhere. The skin over and around the swelling was normal, except where the frequent application of vesicants produced a livid redness. Of the origin of the swelling the afflicted could give no other cause than that he had for a long time, in the spot now occupied by the swelling, a dull, so-called rheumatic pain and that the swelling had grown very slowly to its present size. Of his previous history we learned that while he had never enjoyed good health, he was liable to "catching cold," and had noticed that all his ailments were accompanied by chilliness, which was also true at the present time. All his lesser indispositions presented an irregular intermittent character.

Many years before he had had gonorrhœa, which had continued for an entire year and had been treated in the usual manner, and even now from time to time it appeared, but was of short duration. From this gonorrhœa had come a swelling of the epididymis.

The physical examination of the chest, abdomen and spinal column gave only negative results, while the closest examination by pressure and percussion failed either to produce pain or any condition which might render clearer the puzzling cause of the swelling. It had the appearance of an abscess due to congestion, an opinion which had been given by one of the professors of the faculty. This professor had also advised an exploratory puncture and the opening of the abscess; but this advice the patient had not followed and was led to consult me.

In examining the history and constitution of the patient it appeared to me very reasonable to consider the swelling as a result of a sycotic rheumatoid dyscrasia, and with this view I ordered *Thuja* 30 and *Nat. Sul.* 2x, the former morning and evening and the latter every two hours during the day, and to follow the diet of this constitution. On March 23rd the abscess was smaller, the overlying skin relaxed, the muscular system was in firmer condition, the patient felt much better and the colour of the face was improved. Remedies continued.

On March 31st the abscess had lessened one-half in size and the chronic epididymitis was smaller while the general health of the patient was still improving. Remedies continued. On April 8th the abscess was reduced to a minimum and the epididymitis gone entirely. He was now compelled to return home to resume his duties, but in August I heard from him that he was then in excellent health, all traces of the abscess having disappeared.

Case XVI.

Intermittent with Skin Conditions.—Nux 3x *and* Arsen. 3x, Thuja 30 *and* Nat. sul. 2x, *then* Silic. 3.

M.L., 32, whose sister had been a servant in my house for eleven years, of large size and good constitution, now in her thirteenth year of married life; childless; had when a child and also since her marriage, a scrofulous, oozing eruption on the head and face. She had had only measles out of the list of children's diseases. The menses appeared when she was fifteen. The eruptions on the head were finally removed after the long use of salves and ointments. Soon after this she noticed a small painful induration at the angle of the right lower jaw, which slowly increased in size. In the autumn of the same year, 1867, she was seized with a severe tertian fever with a hard and long-lasting chill, the attack persisting for three months in spite of the use of *Quinine* and other remedies. Immediately after the disappearance of the fever the above-mentioned induration began to enlarge rapidly, became inflamed and suppurated; the latter continued for several weeks with considerable destruction of tissue, leaving an unsightly wound. In the Spring of 1868 she had another attack of tertian fever, which again lasted three months, reappearing again in the Summer for a short time and again in the beginning of July, this attack lasting for one week.

Towards the end of July an eruption of tubercles appeared on the forehead, continually spreading and covered with a thick crust, underneath which was a copious, pus-like secretion. This continued for a long time and left behind a red, irregular, hard, puffy-looking sore. The eruption slowly spread over the forehead and temporal regions and upwards into the hair, and was accompanied by an intolerable itching. At the same time, with this eruption, there began a violent, at times sleep-preventing, dull tearing pain in the right upper jaw, which was < in damp weather and accompanied with swelling which extended up to the eye. This swelling rapidly increased so that by the end of September the right eye could be only partially opened.

The anxiety due to the trouble with the eyes sent her from the country where she had been up to this time, into the next government town, Nishny Novgorod. After a trial of remedies, resection was advised, but to this she would not consent without my opinion. This was in the end of September, 1868. Her condition was now as follows :

Long continued chilliness with flashes of heat ; weak, feeble, emaciated, sallow complexion ; on the forehead the above-described eruption. The swelling of the right jaw was very prominent, almost the size of my fist and reached to a level with the cornea, covering nearly the whole cheek. It felt as hard as a bone, the skin over it was unaltered, moveable and of natural colour and structure. Pressure on the swelling caused no pain. Examination within the mouth showed no alteration of the hard palate. The teeth were in normal position and firmness, but many were carious and nearly all of them blackened, which was due, as the patient said, to severe toothache, which came on like an intermittent, was long continued and suddenly ceased. The space between the eyelids was greatly lessened, and the eye continually watering, a trouble which had affected both eyes since childhood. The vision was distorted ; the pain was described as dull, tearing and greatly < at night and in stormy weather ; no headache, menses regular, no leucorrhœa.

The appetite is fair, stool regular, lungs normal ; no trouble with digestion ; *aversion to fish*, which she cannot look at, to say nothing of eating, *nor can she bear warm or cold baths* since these produce either fever or toothache or pains in the limbs or headache, so that she very seldom, or only for the sake of cleanliness, uses the bath-tub.

Whatever the diagnosis, the eruptions could not be definitely defined, since the spot was covered with a thick crust from beneath which could be pressed in large quantities a purulent watery discharge. The previous attack had left no scarring. In consideration of the papules, the profuse suppuration and the existing bone-swelling I could only conclude there was tuberculous infection with lepra characteristics. The swelling of the upper jaw was diagnosed as an enchondroma. The ground on which this affection grew must, according to all examples, be due undoubtedly to the sycotic-hydrogenoid constitution, and this was confirmed when we knew that the patient had always lived near the Volga, and that in the Spring the high water reaches to the windows, and the land itself was low and boggy. On account of the frequent returns of the intermittent fever, which was not cured, as shown by the still long-continued chilliness, and seeing that it had probably been suppressed by the large doses of *Quinine*, I gave *Nux* 3x and *Arsen* 3x. in hourly alternation of three to four drops each ; also the wine diet and strict avoidance of articles forbidden by the hydrogenoid constitution.

By the middle of October there was general improvement. As I did not expect these remedies to have any marked effect on the eruptions and bone swelling, I gave *Thuja* 30 and *Nat. sulph.* 2x in the same manner as before.

In the beginning of November the eruptions had almost disappeared, there was no discharge, and the itching and reddish discolouration had lessened, while the swelling, at least, had not increased and the pain was very much reduced.

At the end of November the tumour had softened and lessened. On December 12th there was a further change in the tumour but the eruption had entirely disappeared. At this time she was called home and received *Silica* 3, a powder morning and evening. In the beginning of May the patient wrote that all her troubles had disappeared. Anyone who has studied the constitution and has learned to apply the results in practice will be convinced that *Silica* would not have performed so prompt a cure had not its relationship to the diseased constitution been so marked.

CASE XVII.

Hydrogenoid Menorrhagia. Nux *and* Arsen.; Nat. mur.

Madame A. L——, mother of two children, of robust constitution, fleshy, never had a severe illness, menstruation regular and copious until the Autumn of 1867, when her menses came on in an unusually severe form. At first she thought little of it, but as it continued beyond the accustomed time she became worried and consulted me. Careful examination failed to discover any cause for this menorrhagia. The appearance of the flow was about natural, but the quantity had increased to a hæmorrhage. There was no pain, functions of the body normal, and before the onset of the menorrhagia there had been nothing to complain of. Under these circumstances it was not easy to apply a remedy, and one after the other of those prominently indicated for hæmorrhage was tried and failed. *Salina* afforded a passing improvement for one week only. She was nursing her youngest boy and thinking this might be a possible cause it was forbidden. With the onset of Winter, which was a dry and unusually severe one, the menorrhagia ceased. She was neither emaciated nor weak, although the hæmorrhage, with brief interruptions, had lasted two months. During the winter the menses appeared several times in normal quality and quantity. In the early Spring, which was a very damp one, the hæmorrhage returned, and as the patient had lost confidence in homœopathy and myself another physician was consulted. He ordered injections of *Ferrum sesquichlor*, and gave internally *Iron*, *Secale cornutum* and *acids*, but without the slightest relief.

In October, 1868, on my return home after an absence of several months, I was again called to see the patient and learned that *the hæmorrhage ceased on the outset of warm and pleasant weather*, but that *at the beginning of the rains and cold weather*—which was in the early Autumn—the hæmorrhage had again returned and with the same conditions. A most thorough examination failed as before to show the slightest cause for the condition. Noticing now that the attacks *ceased in Summer* and *came on* in the Autumn I asked concerning damp weather or baths, and whether fish, milk and fruit agreed, but to these questions no definite or satisfactory answers were obtained. However, *Nux* 3x and *Arsen.* 3x were given in hourly doses, and the wine and hydrogenoid diet ordered. On the next day the hæmorrhage ceased and remained away two weeks, but returned again after the patient had been out on a very wet day. I strictly forbade going out in similar weather, gave the same remedies and ordered the whole body to be rubbed every morning with brandy. The next day the hæmorrhage ceased and did not return until July, 1869, after she had remained for a long time during rainy weather in a building which was not perfectly dry. During this time the menses appeared in normal quality and quantity and without pain.

The remedies were given at longer intervals and in higher dilutions while the diet remained unchanged. When the hæmorrhage again returned I gave *Natrum mur.* 9, two drops every two hours and after a few days the hæmorrhage was again controlled. A few months later I was informed that she was pregnant.

CASE XVIII.

Sycotic Tumour. Hepar 3x, Thuja 30 *and* Nat. sulph. 3x.

Johann v. T., 37, of strong, robust constitution, a cavalry officer, consulted me in August, 1869, concerning a swelling on the thigh which had existed since 1859, and for the past seven years he had been unable to walk except with the help of a cane, and even then not without limping. The swelling was on the left thigh, almost at the middle, in the rectus femoris muscle, having an eliptical shape and measuring 6½ inches long, 3½ inches broad and 3 inches high. It was slightly moveable, lay embedded between the muscles, was hard and even, feeling like a convolution of a hardened gland and only slightly painful on handling. A portion of the skin covering it was of normal hue ; on the other portion was seated superficial, livid-bluish ulcerations, with a watery, serous, transparent, but at times reddish discharge. A few of the ulcers, of irregular size and varying shape, were cicatrised and had formed dark, dirty blue and livid spots, while others were only apparently covered over, and underneath suppuration was active, discharging through a small fistula. On the side of the swelling towards the knee the ulcers are close together, a few of them in long sinuses extending into the swelling itself, pressure upon which caused a profuse discharge similar to the above. On the lower leg and over the body were numerous livid, blue superficial spots, the results of former furunculi. The pain is not severe but is < by motion and disappears almost entirely by rest. The face had a dirty yellowish colour, but not marked ; the patient was not emaciated, and digestion, appetite and sleep were not disturbed. The limited motion in the limb, especially at the knee-joint, rendered it difficult to bring the joint into more than a very obtuse angle, so that the limping gait was very similar to that caused by disease of the knee-joint. There was pain in the swelling, knee-joint and leg on attempting to bend forwards. Physical examination of the chest and abdomen revealed nothing abnormal; the left testicle was somewhat larger than the right and felt harder but pain was not present.

The general condition, although satisfactory, had, in comparison with his former state, greatly declined. The mind was weakened, spirits depressed, he was easily excited to anger, especially over trifles, which was not the case formerly.

The previous history was as follows: He had never suffered from an acute affection but, on the contrary, had always enjoyed unusually good health. In February, 1855, he had, after an illicit intercourse, a small, slimy, itching sore on the inner surface of the foreskin which healed of itself in a short time. In October, on account of a similar cause, the same sore appeared, was pronounced syphilitic, was treated in the usual manner and healed in a month.

In the Spring of 1856 he was attacked with intermittent fever which continued for several months, showing first a tertian and then a quotidian type. After the fever had been cured with large doses of *Quinine* there again appeared an ulcer following as before an exposure, which was treated with *Mercury* but was slow in healing. The intermittent fever appearing during the period, the *Mercury* was alternated with *Quinine*, and now the ulcer and the intermittent promptly disappeared. A few months later balanitis appeared but was promptly relieved with a lead wash.

In the winter of 1857, the sore which was supposed to have been healed in the previous year again opened, and was healed as before with the sublimate. The ulcer again healed, and in the Summer the patient took on his own responsibility, to cleanse the blood, a so-called "Spring-cure," or *Sarsaparilla* decoction. But in order to secure a sure result he mixed Colbert's essence with the decoction. In the winter of 1858 the ulcer again appeared without apparent cause in spite of the previous prophylaxis; probably the blood-cleansing liquid had not washed it sufficiently. Colbert's essence was given and the ulcer again disappeared to be followed by a balanitis, which was also cured.

Now the patient began to feel weak and exhausted, with falling out of the hair and an uncomfortable feeling of weight in the left thigh, with difficulty in bending the limb, especially at the knee-joint. Later there was an increase in the circumference of the limb. In 1859 he had a left-sided orchitis without apparent cause, and now *Kali iodatum* and leeches joined the series. These benefited the orchitis, but it was followed by a furuncle on the lower leg with long-continued suppuration which was healed with *Muriate of Soda*. To these conditions was added a dry cough, accompanied with retching and continuing throughout the day accompanied each evening with chilliness. This was treated with *Rhubarb and Quinine* pills. The swelling in the thigh now increased rapidly and had in 1863 reached quite a size. In 1865 the trouble had increased still more, notwithstanding the use of *Merc. iod.* and *Sublimate* and other remedies, including baths and ointments, with the result only of producing numerous furunculi over the whole body. Finally, losing all hope of relief, since several consultations of professors had been held over his case, he came to me.

On account of the often-reported, falsely considered syphilitic and mercury mis-treated ulcer, the balanitis, orchitis, furunculi, the characteristic scarrings, the appearance of the same general affections in different organs as well as the intermittents and the characteristic cough, due to the long-continued use of *Quinine*, it was only possible to arrive at one diagnosis, namely, a blood infection on a sycotic or hydrogenoid basis. The swelling on the thigh was also considered a neoplasmus due to the same cause.

There could be no doubt about the preliminary treatment. All salves and ointments were laid aside and dry charpie applied to the suppurating sores, and a wine and hydrogenoid diet ordered. In order to antidote the effects of the *Mercury*, although no salivation had been produced, I gave in August, 1869, three drops, three times daily of *Hepar sulph.* 3x. In September there was a general improvement and now *Thuja* 30 and *Nat. sulph*, 3x was given. In the latter part of October the pains in the leg had disappeared, the swelling had greatly lessened and he was able to move so well that at an evening company he had been able to dance a polka. In December, 1869, the swelling measured exactly 1½ c.m. long and about the same width. All ulceration as well as the hard scars or spots had disappeared. He walked freely without a cane and could move the limb without difficulty in any direction.

The remedies were repeated at longer intervals. I often saw this patient during the following ten years; he had married, was a father and was not again sick.

Concluding Remarks by Dr. Bojanus.

Whoever will take the trouble to compare what is here written upon the causes and character of the disease-relation with what Grauvogl has stated in his writings on "Intermittents" will see that very much of what is there written is here fully confirmed. At the same time he will also see the necessity of asking himself this question—Whether it is possible, without the knowledge and recognition of these constitutions, to cure such cases as safely and in as comparatively a short time with such moderate therapeutic measures?

I am well aware that the history of special cases of sickness is convincing only to those under whose eyes they take place, and who themselves are interested in them in their professional character. This is also to be regretted because of an inviolable law that man never becomes wise by the experience of others but only by his own, if he becomes so at all. We should think and hope, therefore, that in a science like ours, in which three or four lifetimes, if they were allotted to one human being, would not suffice to learn more than a small part of it by personal experience, that the experience of others should at least stimulate examination especially by the more highly educated classes to which physicians belong as well as by those who are advanced in mental culture. And this the more as they put off prejudices and reject them, and when men who on the field of research have made their mark point out doctrines that differ from ordinarily accepted views it by no means follows that they are incorrect or false.

Thus, for example, B. H. Gross, who in matters of science must have more than one voice if his achievements are appreciated, says concerning the doctrines of the constitutions of Grauvogl:

"Grauvogl's fundamental laws have been declared impracticable by men of opposite views, by some out of mere dogmatic habit, by others because they found it too inconvenient to bind their accustomed arbitrary proceedings to study laws. Were they aware how much labour they could save by Grauvogl's works they would study them for their own interest; for the fundamental characters of constitution alone render it possible, to a certain degree, to generalise without becoming unfaithful to homœopathy. As epidemic constitutions they must be very important for the diagnosis and treatment of climatic diseases in all countries of the world. They make it possible to cure with one single remedy a complicated constitutional ailment."

Dr. B. H. Gross quotes the following pertinent Motto. "A physician is he who lays open the wonder-works of God to each and every one. For what is in the sea that may be hidden from the physician? Nothing! What is in the earth that he should not open? Nothing! He shall bring it forth and not alone in the sea, in the earth, in the air, in the firmament! *Requirimus in medico non solum microcosmi sed etram universæ naturalis philosophiæ cognitionnem, non ex phantasmibus ac speculatoribus sed sensuum et experimentiæ judicio exortam.*"

PARACELSUS.

"The doctrine of Constitutions as Grauvogl teaches it in his *Text-book* has found very little favour in Europe, but somewhat more in America; whether justly must be evident by good will to anyone that is free from prejudice."

A RECENT CASE.

To the above record and remarks of Dr. Bojanus I may add a recent case of my own.

A man of 60 who had long been subject to nasal and bronchial catarrh with asthmatic complications, though otherwise well, after some years' residence on high ground, returned to a former residence close to the river. All his old troubles returned in great intensity. On January 1st, 1926, he was put on the double salt of *Mercurius biniodatus* and *Kali iod.* 3x, gr. viii., night and morning. Under this he made great progress for a time, but had a bad relapse in which it ceased to help. An "awful running, sneezing head-cold " came on, leaving congested nose, cough with whitish expectoration, difficult breathing and depression.

I prescribed on January 20th *Ipec.* 3x, discs half an ounce. Two discs to be taken every three hours ; and *Nat. sulph.* 3x, ten grains night and morning. I told him also to confine his baths to one a week, and on the other days to be content with a brisk rub with a rough towel in the morning on rising.

March 4th. Very much better. Still discharge from nose but not so bad. *Repeat.*

March 22nd. He reports : " I am pleased to tell you that I am very fit and that all my old troubles are very trifling."

So he is not thinking of changing his residence again for the present! The medicines were continued.

Chapter VII

THE OXYGENOID CONSTITUTION

Concerning this "Constitution" Grauvogl has more to say than on either of the other two, but he gives no illustrative cases since he considers this unnecessary. Bojanus says he has only seen one typical case of the kind.

As the Hydrogenoid constitution hinders the proper oxygenation of the blood and tissues by a predominant water-logged or hydrogenous condition, so the oxygenoid tends to an excess of oxygen and consequently exaggerates breaking down of hydro-carbons, nitrogenoids and albuminous tissues and bones. We see this in syphilis and its analogue in medicine—Mercury. Thus the oxygenoid constitution corresponds to Hahnemann's Syphilis and also to Bazin's.

This constitution, whether inherited or acquired is of a grave character, says Grauvogl. The blood is a product of the organism and its elaboration is handed down from parents to children for generations. Immunity may also be inherited. A weakened power of resistance against the destructive energy of oxygen may be acquired by attacks of acute epidemic diseases and by syphilitic infection. The incubation periods required by these diseases between the original infection and the outbreak of symptoms is the period required for the increase of the poison up to the degree necessary to make it efficient. These poisons must therefore be living organisms, which induce the most intense processes of reduction, so changing the constitution of the body as to render it unable to resist an immediate influx of oxygen,

It will thus be seen that Grauvogl included under the term "Oxygenoid" much more than is included in Hahnemann's and Bazin's "Syphilis," just as "Hydrogenoids" included more than the results of Gonorrhœa. As for Syphilis itself, Grauvogl believed it quite possible that this poison should arise *de novo* from ferments generated in impure vaginæ and that it depended on the constitution of the individual in question which disease followed from one and the same exposure. "From the same woman on the same day, and indeed in the very same hour, one may get a syphilitic ulcer, one a sycotic ulcer and one escape without any infection." Somewhat parallel with this I have seen a distinct case of syphilis develop in a woman when her partner for months past never had and never developed syphilis; and I have seen a very inveterate urethritis in a man whose wife suffered from leucorrhœa and with whom there was no question of other intercourse. Burnett held much the same view that Grauvogl did, that poisons were generated by the contents of vaginæ of women who had connexion with numbers of different men.

It all depends on the constitution of the recipient, says Grauvogl, which disease is communicated. "Only within and in connection with the Hydrogenoid constitution does the vaginal poison become the cause of the sycotic secretion of the so-called gonorrhœa. It can produce gonorrhœa as well as ulcers ; but these are not cured or benefited by *Mercury*, but aggravated." The sycotic, hydrogenoid dyscrasia follows the suppression of these diseases by injections or by local measures.

On the other hand, the so-called *Chancre-dyscrasia* is produced from the *Oxygenoid* constitution. "Chronic diseases which result from these conditions from the begetting of the *Chancre-poison*" will be cured by *Mercury*, while *Thuja* or *Nat. sulph.*, the hydrogenoid remedies, will aggravate.

Speaking generally on the remedies for the Oxygenoid constitution, Grauvogl says, that on account of too active an influence of Oxygen on the body this seeks its remedies mainly in the Carbon and Nitrogen series which prevent the oxidation of tissues. "Rademacher places *Iron* in the first rank, but I put first Hydriodate of Potash—*Kali iodatum*—because it absorbs all the ozone. Here the carbon and alkalis rich in carbon have a different effect, as *Graphites*, *Petroleum*, *Kreesote*, *Benzoic acid*, *Citric acid*, *Hydrocyanic acid*, *Laurocerasus*, and, chiefly for inductive reasons, Antozone water, corresponding indeed to iodosmone water. Furthermore, *Nitric acid* ; also many co-called narcotics, especially *Aconite*. Moreover, *China*, *Quinine* and *Arsenic* (given alone and not in alternation with *Nux*) ; and also the metals which are capable of suspending the process of decomposition, hence *Chromium* and *Kali bichromicum*."

It will thus be seen that remedies for the Oxygenoid constitution are largely anti-syphilitic remedies as recognised in homœopathy. And Grauvogl expressly states : "*The law of similars must always decide the special indication.*"

Dr. Pascal, in an article contributed to the *Bulletin de l'Homœopathie* on Grauvogl's Constitutions, gives the following summary of the Oxygenoid which may be usefully appended, although it may appear to involve repetition :

In this oxygen predominates, or rather the proteid matters are struck with instability with a morbid facility of division.

Oxidations are rapid though often incomplete. Consumption of tissue arrives more rapidly than in normal conditions of life. Hydrocarbons and albuminoids being rapidly burnt up leave the tissues defenceless against the burning power of oxygen. Oxygenoids are thin and weigh less than carbo-nitrogenoids of equal volume. This provokes the using up of proteid materials and the cellular framework. Scrofula, rickets, infantile atrophy and various states called "anæmia" result from this.

Oxygenoids feel better in an atmosphere saturated with nitrogen and carbon, in the midst of resinous, fatty or empyreumatic vapours.

They refuse easily oxidisable, animal foods, and seek for fats and hydrocarbons which oxidise slowly.

They are *worse* when dryness is changing to humidity, before storms, before and during tempestuous winds and *better* when it begins to rain or snow and the electric equilibrium is restored.

They are *worse* in foggy weather, and when, with a temperate air, mists rise from the forests. This is the opposite of what obtains in the carbo-nitrogenoids with whom fogs, like those of England, provoke melancholy and tendency to suicide.

Nevertheless there is a certain rainy time which *relieves* hydrogenoids and *aggravates* oxygenoids. This is when the air is charged with ozone and the highest points of the mountains are not covered with mists.

In brief, electric disturbances *aggravate*, and electric equilibrium *relieves* oxygenoids.

In the last analysis the phenomena can be traced to a *plus* or a *minus* of atmospheric ozone. Electric attractions polarise atmospheric oxygen and transform it into ozone (oxygen polarised negatively) and antozone (oxygen polarised positively); it is after undergoing this modification that it becomes an effective and energetic oxidiser. Electric disturbances then act as hyperoxidants and this accounts for their aggravations.

However, watery excess enables hydrogenoids to bear hyper-oxidation better, for it demands a still greater storage of heat. This is why rainy weather, charged with ozone, *relieves* hydrogenoids under certain circumstances whilst it *aggravates* oxygenoids.

Other symptoms constantly found in oxygenoids are :

Excessive elimination of urea and phosphates;

Plethora—great quantity of blood ;
Much oxygen fixed on the hæmoglobin ;
Excessive thinness.

Animal heat, strong after meals and feeble in the intervals.

Vigorous appetite which persists astonishingly during illnesses.

Abstinence, on the contrary, is badly tolerated.

> by Rest and Food.

< by Cold, Sea-air, Low altitudes.

Oxygenoids are what are commonly called nervous individuals characterised by great physical and mental activity.

TREATMENT.

Grauvogl puts in the first rank *Kali iod.* since it absorbs all the ozone. Rademacher gives the first place to *Ferrum.*

Among remedies having a direct action on oxygenoids are the *Carbons* and compounds rich in carbon, *Graphites*, *Petrol.*, *Benzin.*, *Citric ac.*, *Hydr. ac.*, *Laurocerasus*, and also, by inference, *Antozonised water*, which is probably equal to Iodosmised water (*l'eau iodosmée*) ; *Nitr. ac.* and a great number of bodies capable of checking the destructive process : *Ars.*, *Chi.*, *Chi. sul.*, *Chrom.*, *Kali. bichr.*

The law of similars always decides special indications.

Chapter VIII

CARBO-NITROGENOID CONSTITUTION

This constitution is characterised by insufficient oxygenation and the diseases it produces are called *diseases of retarded nutrition.* This makes for increased liability to disease and *perverted nutrition.*

After a period of obesity, thinness follows. Albuminoids are decomposed like the hydrocarbons. There is pseudo-albuminaria, phosphaturia, acetonemia, rickets and osteomalachia. *General symptoms* are great frequency of respirations with shallowness ; short breath, frequent pulse, blood charged with melanotic cellules. Constipation or diarrhœa, flatulence, urinary troubles, gouty pains in the head, gouty swellings, vertigo, ataxia, dulness of the head, somnolence, yawning, hypochondriasis, irritability, and extraordinary impatience.

Copious uric acid and oxalates in urine.—Epistaxis and hæmorrhoids.—Pruritus.—Precocious baldness with perspiration of the head.—Cerebral fatigue.—Unhealthy skin, fetid and acid perspiration, boils, eczema, urticaria.

Causes of Aggravation.

1. Everything which hinders oxidation.
2. Everything which increases hydrocarbons and albuminoids.

3. Everything which diminishes the alkalinity of the humours.

< Rest. < Non-ozonised mists.

< Irritation of cerebro-spinal or sympathetic nervous system.

< Sexual excesses.

< Over-feeding.

< Confined air.

< Chagrin.

< Respiratory insufficiency.

< Loss of blood or blood-letting which diminishes the number of blood globules and consequently oxydation.

< Excess of Sodium salts, like sea salt, which hinders cellular osmosis and diminishes the quantity of water in the tissues.

Treatment.

The Cabro-nitrogenoid lacks ozone and is rich in carbon and nitrogen. Consequently it finds its chief remedy in ozone and ozonated water.

Applicable also are all remedies which facilitate the splitting up of hydrocarbons and albuminoids and the discharging of oxygen chemically into the heart of the tissues. For example :

Cupr., Phos., Sulph., Camph., Hepar sulph. Aco., Merc., Aur., Argent., Plumb., Plat., Ol. tereb., Rhus., Dulc., Cham., Lyc., Bov., Bel., Nux. 30 (alone—not alternated as for Hydrogenoids), Digit., Hyos., Apis., Lob. infl.

CHAPTER IX

PRACTICAL EXAMPLES OF THE CARBO-NITROGENOID CONSTITUTION

CASE I.

Dyspnœa, Palpitations, Asthma, etc. Arg. n.

[Symptoms in italics are found in the provings of *Argent. nit.*]

J——. L——., a police officer, 54, complained that for a year past he could no longer satisfy his desire for hunting because, when ascending a hill or on moderately rapid motion *he loses his breath.* He stated that he suffered from piles and had always taken many powders and pills which relieved him, at most, for a day or two, and that now his digestion is so much impaired by having taken them for years, that for many months he has suffered from loss of appetite. Previously corpulent, he was now *emaciated* and has *to complain of a constant anxious feeling in the region of the heart, periodical pains in the abdomen,* burning hæmorrhoidal tumours and *urgency to urinate.* He was most alarmed by the frequent *vertigo and the weakness of the whole of the left side of his body.* He has a prematurely old look, *ashy pale colour of the skin, the tongue was coated white, the taste unpleasant, the region of the liver sensitive to pressure* though no enlargement of the liver could be discovered. No blood or mucus was passed with the stools. Respiration 26, pulse 108; *palpitation of the heart*; no cough, the respiratory murmur scarcely audible in several places; only on the upper part of left lung was it dry, vesicular and manifestly more acute. When requested to draw a deep breath he did it without pain but with so little elevation of the thorax, with so small a quantity of air being inspired, and without being able to hold his breath for any time, that it was clear that the capacity of the lungs was much diminished. *The hands trembled;* the sleep was short and he awoke frequently with *attacks of suffocation.* Discharge of wind upwards and downwards always brought relief. He had lived moderately ever since he could remember.

Soup, meat, vegetables, milk, coffee and two glasses of beer a day were his food. He walked two hours every day in the open air and never smoked.

The use of coffee was forbidden and *Nux vom.* 2 was prescribed provisionally once a day for eight days, then set aside for eight days, and so on.

For eight days he thought he was feeling better, that is, in general only, for all his complaints remained, though in a less degree.

Four weeks later at 2 a.m. he had a violent attack of *asthma*, more violent than ever; this was apparently, according to his statement, caused by cold although it was in the middle of summer. *Arsen.* 10, two or three drops every two hours, was ordered. After three hours he was quiet again, but there was still violent palpitation and short respiration. Arsen. 10 once a day. After six days he returned to his occupation as his breathing had become easier. *Sulph.* 30, a single dose. Better sleep followed and better appetite, and he felt stronger. But after another four weeks he still had no *real inclination* to work, was also tormented with *anxiety*, and, although not so often with vertigo, yet with *confusion of the head and constipation*—the latter always aggravating all his complaints.

For the next six weeks everything remained much the same. But now he earnestly begged for something against the constipation ; for after two or three days without an evacuation there regularly returned intense *weariness* and more *trembling of the hands* ; then also more *sleeplessness and disgust for all labour* ; heaviness and *stupefaction* of the head, especially the occiput ; *eructations* and *sense of constriction in the bowels, as if tightly girt by a band*, which had chiefly set in after the last asthmatic attack. The *urgency to urinate* also increased, while he suffered from obstruction ; also the *palpitation and difficulty of breathing*, as well as the *sense of weakness of the left side of the body, and the left arm became then as heavy as lead.*

Thus *Sulphur* was clearly not indicated, the improvement being too trifling.

In view of the proving of the Carlsbad springs by Dr. Porges, I thought best to advise the patient to take every morning half a teaspoonful of Carlsbad salts in half a pint of water.

This advice was followed for two weeks when, suddenly, for the first time a hæmorrhoidal bleeding ensued with great relief of all his complaints. The relief did not continue long, however. With the spontaneous cessation of the hæmorrhages, during which no remedy was taken, the previous ailments came back. In this way a whole year passed and I had to confess to myself that nothing worth mentioning had been accomplished, although the patient was content.

It is certain that in this case the life of the blood was the primitive seat of attack, and it is equally certain that the insufficient nourishment of the nervous system thence arising proved all these symptoms taking their origin in functional changes in the brain and spinal cord. With this man the entire interchange of substance was impeded by insufficient oxydation, and among those remedies which are able in any way to increase the influence of the oxygen upon the system I found only one which was at the same time indicated according to the law of Similars, *Argent. nit.*

Here, however, let me point out that our patients, whether they take *Arg. nit.* by drops in spring water (for they have no distilled water), or use pellets mediated with *Arg. nit.* and then dissolved in spring water, never really take *Arg. nit.* into their blood, but only Chloride of Silver —*Argentum muriaticum*—and the higher the attenuations are the more certain this is, because all spring water contains no small amount of Chloride of Sodium. If a few drops of the second or even the third decimal attenuation be put into a spoonful of water a white cloud of Chloride of Silver is formed at once. How far this may go is clear from the observation that even the fourth decimal attenuation of *Arg. nit.*, an ounce of it. for instance, clearly presents to the light a reddish-brown cast.

[I may interpolate that although the actual substance may be *Arg. mur.* and not *Arg. nit.*, the *Arg. mur.* is in a nascent state when taken into the system, and the effect may not be identical with *Arg. mur.* otherwise prepared and administered.—J.H.C.]

J.L. was now ordered to take for eight days, night and morning four or five drops of *Arg. nit.* 2x, in a spoonful of water. I prefer to prescribe it in this way because the Chloride of Silver is then always freshly prepared, as had doubtless been the case in the provings.

When J.L. presented himself at the end of the eight days, I was not a little surprised, as soon as he entered the room, by the very decided change in the colour of his face (for he was the first patient to whom I had given this prescription according to the above-mentioned indications). His face had assumed once more the incarnadine pale red colour of healthy men, and he himself declared, with beaming face, that he had never felt as well as he did then for twenty-five years past. This alone proved that increased oxidation of the blood had taken place. Moreover, the pulse had dropped to 90 and the respirations to 22; proof enough of increased capacity of the lungs in accordance with which the patient drew a deeper breath, the thorax expanded more, and the breath could be held for a longer time.

But even the reciprocal action in the nervous system was made evident by the restoration of quiet sleep, often lasting five or six hours, and the disappearance of the "band" round the abdomen, a sure sign of an affection of the phrenic, or diaphragmatic nerve.

I now stopped the medicine for eight days, but nevertheless the improvement continued, the stools became more regular and there was seldom any sign of vertigo. Without further medication of any account the cure continued and for three years thereafter he had no complaints.

Case II.

Headache, Vertigo, Dyspnœa, Palpitation, etc.—
Arg. nit.

A blooming girl of 19, menstruating regularly, suffered for five years without interruption from *pressing pains over the whole head, sometimes only on the vertex, sometimes on the left frontal bone, which were > by firm pressure on the painful parts*, and were ascribed to immoderate dancing in the evening, while the many physicians whose advice was sought had been able to give no relief whatever. On being questioned the patient further states that she suffers from *vertigo* and is *easily tired*, whilst at the same time she is *losing her memory*. On going upstairs her *breathing is hurried* and she has *palpitation of the heart*. The *tongue is coated white*. Appetite and sleep are very good, but she is too *sleepy* during the day; *pains in the stomach* here and there, frequently for weeks at a time, with *nausea and vomiting even.* On feeling the pulse I noticed *a trembling of the hands*; pulse 98; *a burning feeling in the region of the heart*; she can breathe pretty deeply without pain, but *cannot hold her breath long*, and on breathing only vesicular respiration can be heard, yet there is no cough. The urine is pale and poor in solid constituents. Nothing more was to be learned.

After the fourth dose of *Argent. nit*, 2, the girl was relieved of all her headaches and she could afterwards breathe much more easily. Her palpitation was relieved also, and her memory returned in full force, for which an interval of five days only was necessary.

Case III.

Calculous Pyelitis.—Arg. nit.

A woman, 37, of lively temperament and healthy appearance, who was married and had given birth to one child, and had recovered well from her confinement, had suffered during the last three years, without any known cause, from attacks of so-called nephritic colic recurring periodically every three months. Attempts were made to relieve the excessive pains by the applications of leeches to the region of the kidneys on both sides, and by the use of purgatives, and it was only after the patient was reduced to the last degree by this treatment that the pains gradually remitted.

On account of her change of residence I was called in to see her in her last attack and found her in *most acute pains in the regions of both kidneys, the pains extending down the ureters to the bladder.* She was lying motionless on her back, since every motion of her body caused her inexpressible pain, and touching the region of the kidneys increased these pains in the highest degree. She was perspiring freely ; pulse 130 ; she sought by frequent and short breaths to avoid deep inspiration, for this increased her pains insufferably. The urine *contained blood*, *was scanty*, *passed often*, *but only a little at a time and by drops.* It contained a visible sediment of crystallised uric acid and pus, with amorphous gravelly concretions, some as large as half a lentil. The clear urine above the sediment was acid and gave a deposit when heated with nitric acid. Thus it was clear that I had a case of calculous pyelitis to deal with. She begged to have leeches applied, as she had some ready and previously she had always experienced relief from them. But nevertheless, she was afraid to incur the pain of turning on her face, which the application would have necessitated, and so was dissuaded from their use on the promise of receiving relief in some other manner. This I could promise when I prescribed *Arg. nit.* 2, four or five drops every hour.

When I saw her again after six hours she was very grateful to me for such prompt relief and so easily accomplished ; for a quarter of an hour after she had taken the first drops she felt greater relief from her pains than was previously the case under the use of leeches. She was able to urinate at once without hindrance, and more copiously, and she was already lying without pain, yet motionless, because the least motion renewed her pains again. On this account she restrained the urine as long as possible; this has been impossible before, but could now be accomplished with ease.

Next morning the pulse was 80 again, and she breathed as when in health. After eight days no more uric acid crystals were passed, but only small concretions. She showed me one of the size of a lentil, which she had passed without pain, and that was the last sign of her disease, which had lasted three years.

From curiosity I had taken some of the urine on the first day for further examination. Besides what has been already mentioned, it contained no trace of triple phosphates, but the well-known epithelia of the mucous membrane of the pelvis of the kidney. Hence the pus could not have come from the bladder.

Three years have now passed without a relapse.

Case IV.

Hydrogenoid converted by Treatment into Carbo-nitrogenoid and cured with Argent. nit.

A woman, 29, was thought when yet a girl of 15, on account of a pneumonia which she had at that time to be tuberculous on account of her brilliant eyes, white teeth, white, transparent skin, and because absorption of the exudation did not take place in connection with the cough which still continued and the purulent expectoration. Cough and expectoration, however, disappeared spontaneously in the course of a year.

The patient continued apparently well till she married in her twenty-first year, and had a miscarriage. From that time forward all sort of troubles broke upon her—at one time anomalies of menstruation ; at another pains in the ovaries ; now spasmodic cough, palpitation of the heart and symptoms of so-called anæmia. All these, however, were transient, and no medical aid was called in.

Four years after that miscarriage she sought my advice for hoarseness which had already lasted five weeks. A suspicious fluor albus was connected with this, and I gave her *Nat. sulph.* to be taken every three hours. The result was really remarkable, since, even on the second day there was but little of the hoarseness left, and on the third day none at all. The fluor albus diminished and after a fortnight ceased entirely.

Six months later she sent for me in haste on account of a spasm in the chest.

It was a common dry asthma. On the lower part of the left side where she had felt the stitches during her former pneumonia, the sound on percussion was dull and no respiratory murmur could be heard. On the upper border of this spot there was a distinct fine crepitatory mucous rattle. Drawing a deep breath gave pain in the part, and a sound of broncophony was heard. The middle and upper portions of the lung as well as the entire right lung were sound. The cause of all this was a violent mental emotion.

This woman had but little colour in her face and pale lips. She was not much emaciated, but well-formed and slender; had no phthisical appearance; the appetite and sleep were good. The menses have been regular for a long time; rather too copious and followed for a day or two by a mild fluor albus. Her parents, still living, are quite healthy. After her attack of asthma, which lasted half an hour, her pulse stood at 90, and her respirations 21. For eight days one dose of *Phos.* 6 was ordered every day.

Called to see her about a year after I found her suffering again with a violent attack of asthma. She merely complained of want of air and fear of suffocation. Her condition was substantially as before, and as she had been quite well since, except for a few slight spasms of the chest, *Phos.* was ordered again as above. The spasm of the chest ceased, but a great weakness remained, lasting for several days and she remarked that *her whole left side especially was of little use to her.* Objectively there was no anæsthesia to be discovered. She confessed that *she became angry very easily, and whenever she did she always suffered for many days from stitching pains in the affected parts of the chest.* I recommended her to take *Aconite* a few times after every such mental emotion.

A few weeks after this she had *hoarseness* again. Nothing was revealed by the laryngoscope. After taking *Acon.* every hour for three days profuse sweat set in, during which the hoarseness, which she supposed originated from a cold taken when washing, ceased.

Six months later, having been living for a year near the water, she had a *quotidian fever* in the autumn, with increase in the stitches in the side and with cough during the paroxysm. Both disappeared always with the sweat. *Nux.* and *Ipec.* put an end to these attacks in three days; yet only temporarily, for the next summer she suffered a relapse; but now more expectoration which *was clearly puriform, and which was mixed with light blood.* *Chin. sulph.* 3 removed all these symptoms in ten days. It was remarkable that the stitches in the side, the cough and expectoration, at each time, lasted only so long as the paroxysm of the intermittent, and that during this time from the part of the left lung originally diseased, there was a coarse crepitant râle extending to the large bronchi manifest on auscultation.

However, as often as she got angry the chills returned as well as the stitches, cough and expectoration mixed with blood.

The patient could never be persuaded to take care of herself for any length of time, nor would she stay in bed except during the paroxysms of intermittent; and since these attacks of cough produced by passion were not seldom accompanied with *vomiting* also, I gave her *Antim. tart.* 3, which always gave her prompt relief and deliverance from her sufferings; but they always returned again from the same cause.

Another half-year probably had passed, when this woman, in consequence of straining her eyes while sewing was taken with *conjunctivitis* with severe *photophobia.* Besides, I noticed that *the left eye-lid fell further over the bulb than the right.* The pupil of this eye was contracted and reacted less to light. On enquiry she said she had often noticed this before, but it had always passed off by itself as well as the *weakness of sight,* which she had sometimes noticed in this eye when working. As for the rest, the sight of the other eye was very good, neither near-sighted nor far-sighted. But in the twilight or under a clouded sky reading or sewing was very difficult for her because *a cloud was always hanging before the left eye.* The use of the ophthalmoscope was prevented by the pain which the light caused, but I could observe no haziness of the media.

At this time it occurred to me that this woman had lately *lost her strength very much* without, however, losing flesh. Her declarations that she felt *much worse in rest than when walking in the open air,* where she could forget her acknowledged loss of strength, until she was obliged to go upstairs again, which for several years past had almost put her out of breath, was a striking proof that there was increased need of oxidation of the blood. On examination of the chest it was found that the vesicular respiration in all moveable parts of the chest was more acute, and that the sound on percussion had become very clear.

In the last sickness of this woman I was led by a symptom in the nervous system to *Argent. nit.*, namely, by the affection of the left eye. But as the patient had for two days taken *Arg. nit.* 2x, night and morning, she was taken with *such a weakness in all her limbs* that she—and this is saying a great deal for her—was obliged to go to bed, where she frequently fell into a *stuporous condition* with yawning and *a cold shudder over the whole body*, and *lost all her appetite*. On the other hand, the left eyelid was as much elevated again as the right; the pupils in both were equally dilated, and the stitching pains in the left side of the chest had disappeared. Without taking any more *Arg. nit.* all these symptoms had disappeared in two days; the curative effects, however, remained, and simultaneously a marked diminution of the cough had taken place although the sound had not changed until now, after the lapse of three years, and the crepitant râle could be only partially heard on a very deep inspiration.

Since that time this woman has engaged in her occupation without interruption and considers herself and looks perfectly well. This much is sure, that from her previous hydrogenoid constitution a carbo-nitrogenoid constitution had developed in consequence of medical treatment, and the latter is also in the way of improvement as the pulse has even fallen to 70 beats.

The above was written three years after the last dose of *Arg. nit.* had been given and three years later the cure had remained permanent.

Case V.

Duchenne's Locomotor Ataxy.—Argent. nit.

The president of a county court, 45, came to me for a frequent *cough* which was often so violent that he *lost his breath* and for *difficulty of breathing* after somewhat rapid walking by which has face was congested. His face was uniformly pale with pale lips; *white-coated tongue;* pulse 116; *violent palpitation of the heart.* Besides, he complained also of increasing *emaciation.*

While auscultating him I observed, to my no small surprise, that on every inspiration the upper part of the abdominal wall drew in instead of expanding; while expiring on the other hand, it expanded instead of receding. The number of respirations was 21. The inspiration, which was at the same time short, warranted the conclusion that there was a marked diminution of the lung capacity, yet the respiratory murmur was to be heard in all parts of the lungs and no nutritive change in the organs of the chest could be discovered. Only in the large bronchi was there a fine crepitant mucous *râle* to be heard. An effort to breathe deeply took away the patient's breath at once. All this not only warranted the certain diagnosis of *paralysis of the diaphragm,* but also of a depressed innervation of the organs of the chest. As I requested him now to walk with his eyes shut he was seized with *vertigo;* he staggered sensibly in the third step; at the fourth he had to open his eyes quickly in order to seize some object and keep himself up, otherwise he would have fallen to the floor.

This was quite unexpected by the patient and alarmed him greatly, but I was able to assure him that he would be perfectly cured. Thus the cause of all his troubles lay in the *medulla oblongata,* the centre of co-ordination (Duchennes' Locomotor ataxy).

Argent. nit. 2x, five drops night and morning was ordered.

Surprising as it was, I did not hear any more from this man for months when, quite unexpectedly, he came to me again to request my advice for his wife. But how his appearance had changed! His cheeks were fat and red, a perfectly healthy colour, with an evident increase of his whole body; he spoke with such long breaths—a thing impossible for him before—that I was not a little surprised by his silence regarding his restoration to health. Asked how he had been since his last visit he replied that after he had taken that little vial of drops all his former complaints had left him. In confirmation he shut his eyes and walked up and down the room without the least staggering.

Case VI.

Hypochondriasis.—Nux., Arg. nit.

An ecclesiastic, married, a man of learning, sociable and highly esteemed in every respect, had been for five years *melancholy*. He was then 51, and had suffered since his thirty-eighth year from hæmorrhoids which bled every four weeks almost regularly. At the same time he was corpulent, yet on account of an intermittent fever which had been removed by *Quinine* several years before, his liver seemed to have been still more disturbed in its functions, since his skin from time to time had had a yellowish tinge. Except for this he had never been ill, although he had had measles and scarlatina as a child.

He attributed his hæmorrhoids to his sedentary and studious mode of living. His melancholy he ascribed to an undeserved slight which he had met with some five years before. This mental depression soon increased until it became a fixed idea that he was neglected and despised by his family. *His calling became indifferent to him;* he performed his duties, as he said, only mechanically. This man, formerly corpulent, *wasted away from year to year; he became insensible* to all social pleasures and lost all desire for labour. *Finally he gave himself up to the distressing idea that all his undertakings would and must fail.*

When visiting me two years ago he complained in addition to the above of constant *drowsiness by day* and of constant *sleeplessness the whole night through; of weakness of memory,* which frequently did not allow him to find the right word, *confusion of the head, want of appetite, trembling of the limbs,* which could also be seen; of constipation, alternating with diarrhœa, while the previous hæmorrhoidal bleedings had ceased, although the tumours which remained annoyed him very much. He complained moreover of lassitude and weariness of the forearms and legs; and what alarmed him most were frequent *congestions to the head,* a pulsation in various parts of the body, which appeared, however, as a jerking of the muscles, and a constant chilliness. Against whatever I proposed to do for him he had the queerest objections. His respirations were 20, pulse 80 to 84. I finally gave him *Nux.* 6, to be taken once a day till better.

For a whole year I heard nothing more from him. He was sent to a water-cure and came back much more miserable than he went in every respect. Afterwards I was informed that he could no longer perform his duties, and for this reason a substitute had to be appointed. He refused food because, as he said, a man who does not work should not eat; however, when driven by hunger he sought in secret to procure food. He spent the most of his time in bed, and when up it was necessary to use every means to keep him from meeting anyone, for then he wept and assured everyone that he was lost beyond hope for this world, and that no one could delude him in that respect, and no one could reason him out of it. His *weariness and depression* had also reached the highest point.

I desired to examine him personally. What an earth-coloured, emaciated, wretched form of melancholy he presented! Stooping over he staggered when walking, despaired of help from himself or others, constantly complained of *vertigo*, and was utterly bereft of all will power. The ends of his fingers had become numb and his *incessant mental distress* was accompanied with twenty-eight respirations per minute and a pulse of eighty-eight. I had hardly exchanged a few words with him when he fell asleep, but through the night he did not close an eye. Now he complained of *pains in the back* too—drawings in the shoulders; he still had constipation alternating with diarrhœa, *chilliness*, and *cold hands and feet.*

There were no sexual complications as his parents were living and healthy, as well as were his children. The source of the hypochondria in this case was, doubtless, the result of primary carbonisation of the blood which, not removed but constantly increasing, had already extended its reciprocal action on the brain and spinal cord and that with an intensity that nothing more could be expected of *Sulphur*. On the other hand, the phenomena were so similar to those of the proving of *Arg. nit.*, or rather of the *Chloride* of Silver, that four or five drops of the 2x were given night and morning. For three days nothing occurred that I could attribute to the *Arg. nit.* The sleeplessness at night, his fixed ideas, etcetera, pursued him unremittingly, and made him still more desponding, because in the drowsiness during the day, which increased at the same time, he thought he had to recognise an aggravation of his condition. On the night of the sixth day he slept well, and instead of being sleepy the following day he was in uncommonly good spirits ; he talked much more on every subject that was presented to him, and for the first time took part in a social evening gathering of gentlemen. Now I thought it the proper time to suspend the use of the *Arg. nit.*, and the improvement progressed more rapidly than I had ever seen it progress in similar cases without the use of the drug. After fourteen days—fourteen days, I repeat—I sent him home cured. His friends could not contain themselves for astonishment at his fine appearance and the complete cure of his complaints. He resumed his duties without any ill effects and with complete success.

Case VII.

Cardiac collapse, Cough, Ataxy.—Acon., Puls.; Arg. nit.

The president of a court of justice, whose father had died of tuberculosis, suffered from his youth up with a cough with purulent expectoration. After a seton had been placed between the fifth and sixth ribs of the left side, and which he has since worn, the cough became more endurable and lost its malignant character. Still he daily coughed when lying down and on wakening; and on ascending long stairs he had to rest often or he lost his breath.

In his thirty-sixth year, however, his wife observed that he always avoided walking in certain streets. Questioned as to the reason of this he replied that the *sight of high houses always made him dizzy and caused him to stagger*; it seemed to him as if the houses on both sides would approach and crush him. This vertigo disappeared at once as soon as he saw no more high houses, and it was noticed on no other occasion.

After the lapse of several years he was taken with pneumonia, during which much blood was taken from him. He recovered very slowly and when, after two months, he finally endeavoured to leave his bed he was seized with *dizziness* which he could not overcome. He was finally taken to the baths at Kreuth and at length returned to his calling. Yet, in exposure to any exhausting labour he *always had a pain which affected the whole head and which made the letters run into one another when reading.*

When 56 years old he came under my treatment for the *cough* which had never left him since that attack of pneumonia. He was much *emaciated*, looked pale, and had the *sunken features of an old man.* In the upper parts of both lungs there were now large, now small vesicular *râles* ; on the left lower portion none but vesicular and bronchial, and the irritation to cough lay behind the middle of the sternum.

Aconite relieved him of his cough by day and by night so promptly compared with his previous allopathic drugs that he became henceforth a faithful adherent of the system.

On examining the chest I found stenosis and insufficiency of the bicuspid valves, and since the cough was confined again to morning and evening I ordered him to take *Sulphur* 6 once in eight days. He now kept tolerably well for a year.

After this his wife requested me to examine him again. He had been obliged to work very hard and she was now alarmed to see that he *stood and walked unsteadily again*, as often as he thought himself unobserved. Before I had a chance to propose to him an examination, he sent to me a few days later, and his servant said I must make haste as he had left his master pale, breathing heavily and blue in the face as if he were dying. In this condition I found him, lying on a sofa and without any pulse, hardly able to speak, which I also forbade him after he had assured me that he did not know of any reason for this distressing condition. *Pulsatilla* 3 was given. He rallied sensibly from second to second; his pulse, which I had known before to be irregular, returned, and after a few days' rest he was convalescent from a condition which I could only explain as caused by a disturbance in the tract of the Vagus and Sympatheticus, which must have been occasioned by a diminished process of oxidation in the blood continuing for so many years. A long respite followed again and he always relieved himself with *Aconite* and *Pulsatilla.*

He finally came to me, however, unbeknown to his wife, and complained that he could only pursue his calling by the greatest effort of will, and that he would be compelled to ask for a vacation because of incessant vertigo pursued him, compelling him always to go close to houses in order to have something to hold on to. Moreover, the little and ring fingers of the left hand had become *insensible.* He noticed also in the *whole left side of the body an indescribable weakness.*

Now according to what principle was this man to be treated, or was he to be held as beyond treatment? Did he belong to the category of Tuberculosis, of Ataxy, or of diseases of the heart or brain, or where, in the drug-provings even could there be found the truly indicated remedy without considering the concomitant conditions which were also presented therein?

After the patient had taken *Arg. nit.* 2x every two hours for five days he was relieved of the affections of the brain and spinal marrow which had lately renewed their attacks and more violently than ever. Even on the very first day he was able to go to his office without fear of staggering and stumbling like a drunken man. Two weeks later he had lost also the insensibility of the left hand. His complaints of weakness of the left half of the body were heard no more and his respiration was again as free as it ever had been.

CASE VIII.

Hæmoptysis in Hydrogenoid. Constitution changed to Carbo-nitrogenoid under treatment.—Nux., Nat. sulph., etc., *finally* Argent. nit.

A merchant, 37, his parents still living and healthy, had taken part, sound and healthy, in the revolutionary war in Baden as a common cannonier without any bodily injury. When seven years old he had had fever and ague; in his twentieth year he had gonorrhœa, which was suppressed by injections. Apart from these he had never been ill.

In April, 1860, when he was 37, while stooping to pat his dog, he was surprised, being then in the best of health, by suddenly *coughing up blood*, and within the course of half an hour he coughed up a wash-basin full. He had, indeed, for several years past, coughed somewhat every morning without taking any notice of it. This cough, however, with bloody expectoration, had now been diagnosed as hæmorrhoidal congestion and treated with leeches *ad anum* and cathartics, although the patient assured his physician that he had never suffered from piles.

On account of the pulmonary hæmorrhage

itself, which lasted three days, common salt was ordered internally and those purgatives were given daily in the form of pills to force the evacuations which, however, had never been wanting. Four weeks later hæmorrhage recurred, and now for half a year it returned almost every four weeks, sometimes lasting only half a day, sometimes two or three days. After this the hæmorrhage intermitted for four months.

While taking a walk in February, 1861, he suddenly had another violent attack of hæmorrhage, and to the treatment of this attack I was called in.

Of tuberculosis of the lungs or of piles there was no trace whatever. The man had a yellow complexion, was emaciated, very weak and had no appetite since he began taking the pills. Sleep good ; pulse 90 ; respirations 35 ; *stitching pain in the region of the fifth rib on the left side.* In the same place there was a fine crepitant *râle* occupying the space of a florin. He was ordered *Acon.* 3, in alternation with *Arn.* 3, every quarter of an hour. The bloody expectoration steadily diminished from hour to hour.

The next day *Acon.* and *Arn.* were given in hourly alternation and it was two days before all blood had disappeared from the expectorations. Now œdema of the feet ensued.

Thus far the hæmorrhages had always taken place during a longer spell of damp weather, and his condition is even more acutely aggravated when there is a cold rain.

On the sixth day, on account of the loss of blood *China* 3 was given every two hours ; and nourishing food, since his appetite was restored, with wine or wine and seltzer water. The pulse remained the same; the respirations fell to 28. But on the least mental emotion the pulse rose and palpitation of the heart ensued.

The patient assured me that conformably with his excitable temperament his pulse had always been very rapid; that he had always been liable to attacks of palpitation, and that for many years he had been careful not to run upstairs so rapidly as he had been previously accustomed to do. His bowels moved generally every day, sometimes not so often, but always of themselves. As his appetite increased the patient gained strength very rapidly, but on account of his decided hydrogenoid constitution it was necessary that he should take every day from this time forth one dose of *Nux.* 3 and three or four doses of *Nat. sulph.* The œdema of the feet disappeared after ten days.

On May 27th, another hæmorrhage occurred after a fit of passion; *Acon.* and *Arn.* prescribed as above. The hæmorrhage stopped on the second day, and from this time forth I gave *Nux.* and *Nat. sulph.* daily. Rapid improvement followed and the remedies were intermitted. The patient spent every evening in the summer in his usual society whose members could not sufficiently wonder at his healthy appearance after what he had gone through.

On November 10th, after a business journey, hæmorrhage again occurred, but lasted only half-a-day and ceased of itself. *Nux.* and

Nat. sulph. were taken as ordered above on the patient's own responsibility.

On January 27th, 1862, after violent excitement, a new hæmorrhage occurred, but lasted only half an hour.

Notwithstanding these repeated attacks the patient had enjoyed remarkably good health, and congratulated himself on his fine fresh appearance and good spirits. The beat of the heart, however, always kept up to 85 or 90.

In September, on a business journey, he had an attack of *intermittent fever with pulmonary hæmorrhage.* Treated by a homœopathic physician with *Ipec.*, *Quinine* and *Acon.* the patient returned home without loss of strength. *Nux.* and *Nat. sulph.* to be taken again for eight days and omitted for eight days, and so on.

After January, 1863 no further medicine was given since auscultation and percussion could not detect the slightest abnormality ; the patient felt well in every respect and began to grow corpulent.

On June 6th, after a cold taken during a profuse sweat on a hot summer evening, he had a chill. He slept well, however, through the night, but woke in the morning with violent febrile heat, with *headache, stitching pains behind the fifth rib* where the stitches had also been observed during the attacks of bleeding. Every breath, and still more every cough, although he coughed seldom, caused a severe stitch in the place, and the patient hence expected every moment a fresh hæmorrhage. Thus I found him in the morning, bathed in sweat; with face reddened;

pulse 120 ; respirations 40 ; tongue with a heavy yellowish-white coating ; much thirst ; disgust for all food ; was only able to take milk as everything else was vomited up again ; sputa consisting of foamy blood ; crepitating rattling on the seat of the pain ; the percussion note scarcely perceptibly muffled.

The previous attacks of hæmorrhage had clearly arisen from a hydrogenoid soil ; hence I did not hesitate a moment to give *Iod.* 3 every half-hour till the stitching pains remitted and after that every hour.

Up to the next morning there had been no change at all. This striking negative result and the anxiety of the patient to keep himself thoroughly covered since a chill crept over his whole body on the slightest movement, though the room was warm—this in connection with the increased difficulty of breathing, induced me to give *Phos.* 3 every hour.

Up to the third day, contrary to all expectation there was hardly a perceptible improvement. The cough has assumed even a dry spasmodic character, which I had to ascribe to the influence of the *Phos.* The sputa were rust-coloured, containing air bubbles of large size, and were scanty. Pulse, respiration, temperature of the skin and perspiration and the results of ausculta-tion and percussion were as on the first day.

To be frank, I did not know any longer what to think of the case, so I gave *Sacch. lact.* in order to gain an undisturbed observation. And I opened the windows *since the patient very earnestly longed for fresh air.*

June 11th. The same state of affairs and *sensible emaciation and wasting of strength.* The sputa had become yellow, but certainly not coloured with "bile-pigment" (!). *China* 3 every two hours was ordered.

June 13th. Less pain, at least, but permanent fever. The patient spoke confusedly and did not know his wife; slept no more; when he talked his speech was broken and he gasped for breath after every word. *Phos. acid* 6 every two hours given.

June 15th. The fine crepitant *râle* became coarse and extended higher. Sputa puriform.

June 19th. Some relief as the cough was less frequent and the respiration more quiet. The sensorium became free again. Up to this time milk and sugar water only were desired. To the former Seltzer water was now added.

The effect of medical treatment amounted to just about nothing; nevertheless the *Phos. ac.* was continued.

June 21st. The appetite was somewhat improved and now and then mucilaginous broth was taken. The urine constantly presented the usual sediment of uric acid, and the stools occurred at first daily; later not so often, though nothing was given on that account. The strength seemed to increase. No further remedies.

June 25th. *Irresistible inclination to get out of bed and sit by the open window.* Now in the armchair—now in bed again. The coarse crepitant *râle*, the puriform expectoration, the cough, the fever, the pain on the side were still present though in a less degree.

June 27th. In addition to the other symptoms he was still *hoarse*. On the other hand he was able to remain somewhat longer out of bed, though it was impossible for him to walk without holding on to something with both hands ; he was altogether too weak to stand erect. *Every time he sat by the window he felt much refreshed.*

June 30th. The fever is sensibly consuming his strength ; his tongue has a *yellowish-white coat*, although he has more appetite ; the urine full of uric acid ; pains in the calves often torment him the whole night, and during the day he is constantly tormented with *formication* in the arms and legs. The pains in the left side of the chest still continue, only they are somewhat deeper and are not any longer increased by coughing ; œdema of both feet. My fear that I should lose this patient by reason of his hectic fever seemed justified ; yet I auscultated him again and found that the coarse crepitant *râle* was limited to the same spot behind the fifth rib, but above, was more extensive, while the pain now was pointed out as corresponding to the sixth rib, which also was painful on being pressed upon as far as towards the spinal column.

I should have been very happy if I could have obtained an anchor, a compass and a helm from the physiological school, since this patient had become a convert to homœopathy under my treatment. But the physiological school had neither for this case, nor for an infinitude of other cases, any pilot.

I had nearly lost this man from disregarding the change which had taken place in the state of his body by reason of the treatment followed for so long a time. First, the circumstance that the pains in the side now correspond to the sixth rib and no longer to the fifth ; that the patient now, on being questioned, declared the present pain to be quite different from what it was at first ; moreover, *his longing for fresh air*, which was never so marked before, the indifferenee to moist or damp weather, observable even before his last illness ; his eorpulence which of late had sensibly increased again. All these went to prove that the hydroscopic condition of his blood was removed; that, on the contrary, its oxidation, even before this last illness was depressed, and during the illness so sank that the spinal cord began to suffer under it, which condition was clearly connected with this *intercostal neuralgia*, the cramp in the ealves, and the *formication.*

Argent. nit. 2x was now given every two hours and the course of the disease after its exhibition is extremely interesting and to the patient himself appeared really mysterious.

Although I never allow a remedy to be taken during the night, very rare cases excepted, and did not in this case, yet the patient declared on the very next day that the pains about the sixth rib, which had affected him so seriously, had become so trifling that they hardly troubled him at all ; also that he had not for many weeks slept so long or so quietly, and had more appetite again. But the most remarkable thing was the daily decreasing crepitant *râle* and the corresponding decrease of the cough and the purulent expectoration. The patient took a new lease of life, and after taking the remedy for seven days the pulse had sunk to 80 and *Argent. nit.* was laid aside.

The convalescence from this all-but-fatal illness progressed with great strides, and by the end of August this man was perfectly cured. He had regained his previous fresh complexion, his good spirits and his mental and bodily strength, returned to his occupation and remained well.

Case IX.

Enuresis with Rapid Pulse. Quick Pulse and Need of Air.—Arg. nit.

A young man, 18, of sound parents, had suffered from his youth with *incontinence of urine*, and after all sorts of tortures had to leave the institution in which he had been a pupil for four years, being declared incurable. In his childhood he had often had swollen glands. Now he is large, powerfully built and I observed nothing abnormal about him except that his pupils were large and that the *beat of the heart* was somewhat more frequent than normal and rather *weak*. He had never suffered from worms and there was nothing peculiar about the constituents of the urine.

Was the indication in this case to direct the patient to retain his urine during the day as long as possible ? Or, should I rather give him Bell., Puls., China, Causticum, Sepia or Sulphur, and on what grounds ?

I gave him instead *Argent. nit.* 2x, night and morning, for six days, and then stopped it. From the first day of taking the medicine he did not wet the bed for a period of six weeks. He had then resumed his studies and was obliged to pass the entire day within four walls. It was certainly an unexpected event that after this day he should wet the bed again. *Arg. nit.* was again ordered and the patient was directed to walk in the open air at least an hour every day, whatever the weather might be. After ten days the incontinence ceased and returned no more.

CASE X.

Malarial-ataxy.—Arg. nit.

A large, powerfully-built merchant, 41, always healthy, had two years before, while travelling, contracted intermittent fever which was suppressed with large doses of *Quinine*. Since then he had never been well, whilst previously he had never been ill, and always had a blooming appearance. A year ago he was taken with gastric fever which had become typhus, as his physician told him. There was no unconsciousness, however, and no hallucinations, no diarrhœa or chest trouble, only constant pains in all parts of the head, especially the occiput, which deprived him of sleep, and every evening he had fever.

These pains in the head finally extended to the eyes and the lower jaw. *Itching pustules* also formed *over the left shin bone, one of which developed into an ulcer.*

After six weeks of allopathic treatment, during which he constantly got worse, lost flesh and all his appetite, he was *so much unstrung and irritated* that, without the knowledge of his physician, he sprang up to get into the open air. Although punished for this by utter prostration of strength, so that he had to ride home, he had to his great delight the first good night's sleep and thereupon more appetite, and that suggested to him the idea that he was not being managed well.

When he came under my care this man, once so corpulent, was so *emaciated* that his clothes hung on him as on a clothes-horse. *At the same time his face was sunken, colourless, and he complained of constant boring headache, and photophobia and weakness of sight, which alone would have* prevented his writing his name legibly, had he not been also hindered therefrom by *trembling of the hands*. Furthermore, he reeled so from *vertigo* at night and when his eyes were closed that he always had to hold on to something. To fix his thoughts on anything, or to *give his business any consideration was impossible ; on attempting it, it immediately got dark before his eyes and the headache increased. Moreover he could not separate his jaws wide enough to admit more than a quill*. That prevented his speaking and he could only take fluid food. But what distressed him most was a disgusting odour from the *little ulcers* with which the inner nose was lined, fearing as he did that those around might be annoyed by it, which, however, was not the case. The stools were regular, the *voice hoarse ;* no change could be discovered in the chest organs by auscultation or percussion; yet the impulse of the heart was very strong and audible over the whole thorax ; pulse 98. The fundus of the eyes was obscured and the vessels could not be seen. Sometimes there was hæmorrhoidal flow but no piles. The fever in the evening was no longer very perceptible, but it seemed to him that he had a fever in his sleep. Since he was taken ill he had never been able to go upstairs without increase of the *difficulty of breathing.*

Whoever has read Dr. Eisenmann's work on *Locomotor Ataxy* will have no difficulty in placing this case under that head, but where, from that work, could a remedy be found ?

This patient also after the lapse of two months was relieved of all his sufferings by the use of *Arg. nit.* He took it for eight days night and morning and then omitted it for eight days, and so on, without the appearance of any drug symptom. After the sight was restored, the nose cured and the trembling of the hands, after it became easier for him to go upstairs, there still remained an insufficient movement of the lower jaw, and I hoped that the secondary effect of the remedy, or rather allowing it to complete its effect would remove this also. It continued, however, for half a year longer, and the staggering when the eyes were closed was still present though in a much less degree. *Arg. nit.* was now repeated. After eight days there was marked improvement. No further remedy was given and after two months the cure was complete.

This was clearly a case of malaria-ataxy, the malaria being the primary cause. We homœopaths have not only *Arg. nit.*, *Arsen.* and *Iod.* as problematical remedies for locomotor-ataxy, but as tried remedies Arg. nit. (or, rather *Arg. mur.*), *Am. mur.*, *Sul.*, *Arsen.*, *Bell.*, *Cyclamen*, *Mangan. acet.*, *Gratiola*, *Phos.*, and *Phos. ac.*

Case XI.

Amblyopia, Blood-rushes, Ataxia. Aggravation and then cure with Arg. nit.

A near-sighted Treasury officer, who wears concave glasses, 51 years of age, had cholera in Munich and subsequently abdominal typhus (enteric). During the past winter he suffered from facial neuralgia and swelling of the bones of the right foot. At the same time *an herpetic eruption was observed on the occiput.* The more this increased the less were the pains in the face, and in the spring they ceased entirely. The eruption also gradually disappeared. On the other hand, in the month of March there was determination of blood to the head, which was treated with *Sulph.* and did not return. During a leave of absence, however, those congestions returned in a very distressing manner. In the course of an hour they were repeated four or five times after they had always ceased spontaneously. He then suddenly felt how the blood pressed from the heart to the head, which became blood-red the colour extending to behind the ears, even. Gradually the blood ebbed again and sweat appeared on the head. These rushes of blood acted injuriously on the eyes. *Since their occurrence objects appeared as if enveloped in a mist; sometimes they seemed double.* After a forced walk these *rushes of blood came also at night;* there was a stitching pain then from the right into the left ear, as if from a thrust with a dagger. In the dark he cannot walk without reeling and laying hold of whatever he can.

Nausea now followed these repeated attacks, and, called to see him once at night in such an attack, I gave him *Bell.* 3 the next morning. This was followed by *confusion of the head,* which was a sign that *Bell.* was not indicated. He can read with his glasses only No. 13 of Jaeger's test letters; the fundus of the eye is injected; the large blood-vessels are indistinct.

Reviewing this case, I must acknowledge that if in Therapeutics there was not a synthesis on the basis of natural laws, a mere analytical comparison between these groups of symptoms and the provings without a consideration of accompanying circumstances could hardly lead to an indication which could foresee the result.

In the group of symptoms just laid down the point of departure of the disease is a more or less diminished influence of oxygen upon the organism.

The patient now received *Arg. nit.* 2x, morning and evening; but after the first day not only was there no improvement but his power of vision was so greatly disturbed that he greatly feared he would lose his sight altogether. He could only read Jaeger 17, and this alarmed even me not a little. *Sacch. lact.* was now ordered. A week later he was able to read No. 13 again. Thus the aggravation from *Arg. nit.* subsided spontaneously without antidoting. Eight days afterwards the condition was as at first. I now ordered *Arg. nit.* 10x morning and evening.

Four days later he returned with the assurance that he could now see better than ever before and could actually read with his glasses, Jaeger No. 4 without difficulty, although with the ophthalmoscope I could discover no change in the fundus oculi.

On the other hand he had felt the good effect of these drops almost instantly; he thought he could distinctly feel the blood settling down from his head. I now directed him to set the drops aside, and some weeks later he called again to say that the congestions, which he noticed for a few days longer, had now entirely ceased and he considered himself quite cured.

The forms as well as the number of diseases in which *Arg. nit.* has accomplished a cure for me are far greater than in the cases here recorded. The forms extend to most of the diseases included in this bodily constitution and even to special diseases of adults and children, including one form of hydrocephalus. The sphere of *Argent. nit.* is so comprehensive because it stands, like *Manganum*, midway between Sycosis and Psora, and is all the more valuable because complications of these two constitutional characters are not infrequent.

Chapter X

CONCLUSION

Von Grauvogl's book contains many other precious gems of practical experience which might be included in this volume, but as they have no direct bearing on the subject of the Constitutions I prefer to let the record of the latter stand out in their clearness unmixed with other topics. Without having encountered many cases as clearly defined as those of Grauvogl and Bojanus, I can say that very few days of practice pass over me without my making some use of the doctrine of Constitutions as here laid down.

According to Grauvogl the human race can be divided into two sections—the born *analysers*, and the born *synthetisers*. But the Homœopath should be born *both*; and if he is only one should make himself the other, whichever he is. It seems to me that the School of Kent have reached the limits of possibility in analysis in the tracking down and matching of individual symptoms. This has been made possible mainly through the monumental work of Dr. Kent himself in his great *Repertory*. But the no less important synthetic work of putting the items of drug symptoms together and finding the connecting thread which runs through them and binds them into an organic whole must not be neglected. Hahnemann himself saw the necessity of this, and the outcome of his research in this direction was his work on "The Chronic Diseases."

Von Grauvogl followed Hahnemann's lead, but struck out an original line of his own. It is one of the grand traits of Homœopathy that it fetters no man's mind. Like Hahnemann himself Grauvogl was an expert chemist and could follow the chemical changes taking place in the blood and tissues. This led him to find new threads and new methods of finding the generalities amidst the particulars. It is not too much to say that his discovery has been more fruitful of results from the prescribers' point of view than any of the others.

Since the day of Hahnemann and Grauvogl the bulk of the Materia Medica has increased enormously and the prescribers' field of choice has increased in proportion. Hence the added necessity of making all possible use of such general indications as are available. As a matter of fact every practitioner does this more or less instinctively, keeping of course, the Materia Medica and Repertory at hand for confirmation of the indications when needed.

That there are various avenues by which the same remedy may be found by different men and different systems is a saving clause in medical practice. But by whatever avenue a medicine is reached, it will act in its own way regardless of the man who prescribes it. The remedies themselves care nothing for systems and theories —they do their own work when brought in contact with it, whether they are given by a

Hahnemann, a Schüssler, a Rademacher, or a Grauvogl.

In my own practice I invariably put to my own patients the same questions that Grauvogl did, and this at once sorts them into sections and narrows the choice of remedies. I also follow the Paracelsic maxim and find, if I can, the *beginning*. If I learn that a patient has never been the same since an attack of influenza either of recent or ancient date, I am fairly certain that a course of the *Tuberculinum of Koch* will be required. If, again, there is a history of vaccination, "successful" or otherwise, in the case, *Thuja*, *Vaccininum* and *Variolinum* are at onee visible in the field. So that there are many other constitutional indications to be found independently of those supplied by Grauvogl. These every practitioner will be able to find for himself.

That the names of diseases are mere abstractions Hahnemann and Grauvogl were constantly insisting. In this they again followed Paracelsus' lead. According to him diseases or morbid states should be called by the names of their remedies. As the Homœopath says "this is a *Lycopodium* case, and that other a *Sulphur* case," Paracelsus writes: "If we say this disease is a disease of *Pulegium*, this one of *Melissa*, that one of *Sabina*, then we have a certain cure from the name. A natural and true physician says that this is a *Morbus Terebinthinus*, that is a *Morbus Helleborinus*, etc.; not that this is *Rheuma*, *Coryza*, *Catarrh*. These latter names do not proceed from curative knowledge; for similars must be compared with similars in names; from this comparison proceed the cures."

The "Pocket-Book" of von Boenninghausen is the most successful work we have in the way of repertorising the generalities of the Materia Medica, and its author has laid Homœopathy under an obligation no less great than that of Grauvogl. It is all in the direction of unifying the great mass of individual symptoms. A further great aid to simplicity in prescribing is that advocated by Dr. Lippe and his friends. Out of the characteristic symptoms of the remedies they marked out those which they named "Key-Note symptoms." Indeed, some symptoms or conditions of symptoms are so characteristic of certain remedies that when one of them appears in a patient it is almost certain that other symptoms of that remedy will be found in the patient too.

Paracelsus wrote: "That which is perceptible to the senses may be seen by everybody who is not a physician; but a physician should be able to see things that not everybody can see. There are natural physicians and there are artificially made physicians. The former see things which the latter cannot see, but the others dispute the existence of such things because they cannot see them. They see the exterior of things, but the true physicians see the interior. The inner man is the substantial reality; while the outer one is only an apparition; and therefore the true physician sees the real man and the quack sees only an illusion."

Said J. C. Burnett: "I don't look where you

look; I let my imaginations play about a case." It was by such "looking" and such play of his imagination that Burnett was enabled to see a nexus between the ringworm parasite and the bacillus of tuberculosis, and which further led him to cure many cases of ringworm with *Bacillinum* or *Tuberculinum*, which in his day was not to be found in Materia Medica or Repertory.

William Blake, who was no physician, but who was a Seer, wrote: "My business is not to argue and compare; my business is to create." And again: "I must create a system for myself, or else be the slave of some other man's." "*Non sit alterius qui suus esse potest*"—"Let him who has power to be his own not be the property of any other man"—is Paracelsus' way of saying the same thing. It is the glory of Homœopathy that it permits everyone to follow his own genius in perfect freedom without fettering him to any man's dictum or authority, be it Hippocrates', Hahnemann's, Grauvogl's, Burnett's, or Kent's. In the last resort every physician must and does create his own system from his own experience, and from such experiences of others as he is able to digest and make his own.

Other men's works provide the nutriment required by the beginner for forming his own mental organism before it can be hatched out of his own experiences. Those who can put their experiences into such shape that others can appropriate their teaching and make it live again, are the greatest benefactors to medical science and art.

It has been my aim in compiling this volume to put the work of one of the chief of these benefactors into such apprehensible shape that all may partake of the feast he has provided and make so much of it as their own genius can absorb a living part of themselves.

INDEX